Masterful Care of the Aging Athlete

Vonda J. Wright • Kellie K. Middleton
Editors

Masterful Care of the Aging Athlete

A Clinical Guide

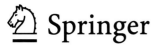 Springer

Editors
Vonda J. Wright
UPMC Center for Sports Medicine
Pittsburgh, PA
USA

Kellie K. Middleton
Department of Orthopedic Surgery
University of Pittsburgh
Pittsburgh, PA
USA

ISBN 978-3-319-16222-5   ISBN 978-3-319-16223-2   (eBook)
https://doi.org/10.1007/978-3-319-16223-2

Library of Congress Control Number: 2018946804

This Springer imprint is published by Springer Nature, under the registered company Springer International Publishing AG
The registered company address is: Gewerbestrasse 11, 6330 Cham, Switzerland

Preface

As an orthopedic surgeon, researcher, and healthy aging advocate, I've seen proof that we all have the power to transform our health through mobility and smart nutrition. In fact, more than 70% of our health trajectory is controlled by the active lifestyle decisions our patients make. Restoring their mobility via conservative and operative intervention is not just a procedure for us to complete, but in the larger scope of our patients' health, allowing them to stay mobile, we are restoring the key to healthy aging.

At ages historically dedicated to "slowing down," masters athletes and active people of all ages and skill levels fill the roads, playing fields, and sporting venues, harnessing the power of mobility and sport to keep them youthful both physically and mentally. Their efforts are supported not only by enthusiasm for active aging, but also by a powerful body of literature that points to mobility as a key element in prolonging health and diminishing the effects of chronic disease and passive aging.

Today, it is common for professional athletes once considered "past their prime" to make significant contributions to their teams and for individual endurance athletes to win events outright at ages pushing 40. These feats of skill, strength, and endurance are not isolated to the professionals alone but reflect a generation who expect high performance from their bodies and prove that our bodies are dynamic adaptors capable of more than we historically have expected of them.

One of my favorite sports writers, John Hanc, in an article for *Best Life Magazine*, summarizes it well:

> It's as though 21st century professional athletes and weekend warriors are living out the Benjamin Button fantasy: Through a combination of scientific training, disciplined diet and advanced sports medicine they are overturning immutable laws of biology and they are reversing or at least fighting to a at draw, the aging process. The new old pros are busy making 40 the new 30. The truth behind the headlines, while encouraging, is complicated. Overall, athletic performance clearly declines with age. At the same time, late-career athletic productivity is showing an unprecedented rise.

As gatekeepers of mobility, the orthopedic surgeon and musculoskeletal colleagues play a key role in keeping these actively aging athletes on the road and out of the doctor's office. This takes a paradigm shift within our own ranks from simply advising people to "slow down and act your age" when injured to an exploration of the clinical, technical, and research avenues for prolonging the ability of masters athletes to optimize their performance and while minimizing injury.

This book is a compilation of clinical, technical, and research approaches to keeping active people moving, returning them to sport rapidly and durably, and protecting them from the sedentary lifestyle that can ravage health.

I am thankful to all my colleagues who join in the movement to save lives by saving mobility and have contributed so heavily in this book.

Pittsburgh, PA, USA   Vonda J. Wright, MD, MS

Contents

Contributors

James Bradley, MD Department of Orthopaedic Surgery, University of Pittsburgh Medical Center, Pittsburgh, PA, USA

Monique C. Chambers, MD, MSL Department of Orthopaedic Surgery, University of Pittsburgh Medical Center, Pittsburgh, PA, USA

Edward Chang, MD Inova Health System, Alexandria, VA, USA

Brian J. Cole, MD, MBA Departments of Orthopedics and Surgery, Rush OPH, Shoulder, Elbow and Knee Surgery, Cartilage Restoration Center at Rush, Rush University Medical Center, Chicago, IL, USA

Jared Anthony Crasto, MD Department of Orthopaedic Surgery, University of Pittsburgh Medical Center, Pittsburgh, PA, USA

Ron DeAngelo, MEd, CSCS, LAT, ATC, FAFS UPMC Sports Medicine, Pittsburgh, PA, USA

Mitchell S. Fourman, MD, MPhil Department of Orthopaedic Surgery, University of Pittsburgh Medical Center, Pittsburgh, PA, USA

Nicole A. Friel, MD, MS Rush University Medical Center, Chicago, IL, USA

Robert J. Goitz, MD Department of Orthopaedic Surgery, University of Pittsburgh Medical Center (UPMC), Pittsburgh, PA, USA

MaCalus V. Hogan, MD Foot and Ankle Division, Department of Orthopedic Surgery, University of Pittsburgh Medical Center, Pittsburgh, PA, USA

Paul Hong, MD Sutter Medical Group Neurosciences, Sacramento, CA, USA

James Irvine, MD Department of Orthopaedic Surgery, University of Pittsburgh, Pittsburgh, PA, USA

Jay V. Kalawadia, MD Department of Orthopaedic Surgery, Orthopaedic Associates of Allentown, Allentown, PA, USA

Brian A. Klatt, MD Department of Orthopaedic Surgery, University of Pittsburgh Medical Center (UPMC), Pittsburgh, PA, USA

Dukens LaBaze, BS Department of Orthopaedic Surgery, University of Pittsburgh Medical Center, Pittsburgh, PA, USA

Drew A. Lansdown, MD Rush University Medical Center, Chicago, IL, USA

Joon Y. Lee, MD Department of Orthopedic Surgery, University of Pittsburgh Medical Center, Pittsburgh, PA, USA

Albert Lin, MD Department of Orthopaedic Surgery, University of Pittsburgh Medical Center (UPMC), Pittsburgh, PA, USA

Jeff Lucchino, MS, RD, CSSD, LDN, CPT UPMC Lemieux Sports Complex, Pittsburgh, PA, USA

Christopher L. McCrum, MD Department of Orthopaedic Surgery, University of Pittsburgh, Pittsburgh, PA, USA

Kellie K. Middleton, MD, MPH Department of Orthopaedic Surgery, University of Pittsburgh Medical Center, Pittsburgh, PA, USA

Chinedu Nwasike, MD Department of Orthopedic Surgery, University of Pittsburgh Medical Center, Pittsburgh, PA, USA

Michael J. O'Malley, MD Department of Orthopaedic Surgery, University of Pittsburgh Medical Center (UPMC), Pittsburgh, PA, USA

Jesse Raszeswki, MBS Alabama College of Osteopathic Medicine, Dothan, AL, USA

Brent Schultz, MD Department of Orthopaedic Surgery, University of Pittsburgh Medical Center (UPMC), Pittsburgh, PA, USA

Farah Tejpar, MD Cleveland Clinic, Weston, FL, USA

Vonda J. Wright, MD, MS Department of Orthopaedic Surgery, University of Pittsburgh, UPMC Lemieux Sports Complex, Pittsburgh, PA, USA

Zaneb Yaseen, MD Department of Orthopaedic Surgery, Cayuga Medical Associates, Ithaca, NY, USA

Philip Zakko University of Pittsburgh Medical Center, Farmington, CT, USA

Emily Zhao, MD Department of Orthopaedic Surgery, University of Pittsburgh, Pittsburgh, PA, USA

Jason P. Zlotnicki, MD Department of Orthopaedic Surgery, University of Pittsburgh Medical Center (UPMC), Pittsburgh, PA, USA

Part I
The Science of Musculoskeletal Aging and the Benefits of Being a Masters Athlete

Chapter 1
The New Science of Aging

Vonda J. Wright

Never in the history of the mankind has there been a better time to age. The mean lifespan at the end of the last century ended in the mid-30s and has risen to nearly 80 years with the implementation of public health and safety initiatives, vaccines and today's medical discoveries for disease treatment.

Today as we look forward expectantly to lifespans maximizing at 114 years, there is a health pivot from disease care to prevention of chronic disease through lifestyle, performance optimization and clinical implementation of exponential technologies that have, until now, been the subject of science fiction.

Much of what we historically know about the aging process came from National Institute on Aging's (NIA) Baltimore Longitudinal Study of Aging that began in 1958 and followed more than 3100 people over time. That study revealed that aging is not a linear process that manifests the same way in every person but instead is as individual as our fingerprints and controlled by the lifestyle choices we make.

Arguably one of the most important lifestyle influences in aging is mobility. The human body was designed for mobility with the strongest muscles in the body anchored through our pelvis and into our legs. Architecturally, it follows that if we were designed for sedentary living, we would have wide immobile bases like mushrooms.

Mobility influences health from macro-level muscles and bones, the microscopic metabolic pathways it stimulates and most importantly, mobility stimulates the genomic and biomic transcription of genes that prevent disease and sustain life.

As orthopaedic surgeons and musculoskeletal clinicians, we are the gatekeepers of mobility with the potential of our work to profoundly influence our patients'

V. J. Wright, MD, MS
Department of Orthopaedic Surgery,
University of Pittsburgh, UPMC Lemieux Sports Complex,
Pittsburgh, PA, USA
e-mail: vonda.wright@northside.com

© Springer International Publishing AG, part of Springer Nature 2018
V. J. Wright, K. K. Middleton (eds.), *Masterful Care of the Aging Athlete*,
https://doi.org/10.1007/978-3-319-16223-2_1

mobility and therefore their health. We are not carpenters, but through restoring mobility, we are preventers of chronic disease and the influencers of active aging.

DNA Is Not Destiny

From the minute of conception to the minute of our deaths, nothing is more natural than aging. Recently, our understanding of this process has changed from a belief that there was nothing we can do to influence the process to an understanding that we can shape our gene trascription via choices we make. This hope is based on the discovery of telomeres, the DNA caps at the end of chromosomes that are known to protect genetic material from damage. With each cell division, usually 50–70 per cell lifespan, the telomeres shorten, and with the shortening come age-related diseases. When the telomeres become too short, the cell can no longer divide and will die.

Recent studies show that mobility and smart nutrition can change telomere length and thus shape aging. A landmark study in Lancet Oncology found prostate cancer patients who implemented positive lifestyle habits including regular mobility, smart plant-based nutrition, mindfulness practices and quit smoking increased their telomere length more than 10% over 5 years when compared to sedentary controls. The more subjects strictly adhered to the mobility and nutrition regimen, the more length their telomeres obtained.

Multiple lifestyle factors including mobility, nutrition, BMI management, moderate alcohol intake and not smoking seem to work in concert to protect telomeres and thus influence aging. In a Harvard study of more than 5000 women, these 5 lifestyle habits practised in concert resulted in dramatic telomere increased on >30%, while habits practised individually had little effect.

Aging and Inflammation

A profound influencer of aging is inflammation. Though designed as a protector against microscopic predators and injury, the healthy inflammatory response lasts only a few hours or days. The orthopod's battle is usually against chronic inflammation of the joints, tendons, ligaments and muscles that persists past the point of healing resulting in cytokines generated during the acute response travelling throughout the body to cause damage to vessels and organs far from the original injury site. Chronic inflammation is a common denominator in diseases of aging including arthritis, diabetes, Alzheimer's, and cardiac disease.

Patient's weight, due to their sedentary lifestyle, plays a significant role in inflammatory aging. As fat cells grow larger, they increase their production of cytokines including IL-6 (interleukin-6). These cytokines block normal metabolic pathways in and out of cells and contribute to insulin resistance and the diseases that result.

Musculoskeletal Aging and Mobility

Slowing down with age is seen across all species from insects to mammals and at all levels within an organism. At a cellular level the regenerative capacity of individual cells decreases and culminates in the macro-level changes we see in organ function, tendon stiffness and joint range of motion. Are these changes in athletes purely due to the biology of aging or due to decreased effort, activity or cumulative injury sequel?

To answer the fundamental question of "what is the aging musculoskeletal system capable of when sedentary living is taken out of the equation", the Performance and Research Initiative for Masters Athletes (PRIMA) at the University of Pittsburgh began a series of studies to evaluate the question in masters athletes who maintain the highest levels of functional capacity and quality of life throughout their lifespans free from the variable of sedentary living and disuse.

Performance as a Biomarker of Aging

Aging-related rates of decline in performance among elite senior athletes were evaluated in runners participating in the Senior Olympic Games Track events from 100 to 10,000 m (Fig. 1.1). Performance times were compared across events and age divisions to determine at what age slowing down occurred. Athletes 50–85 were included with the times of the top 8 finishers in each age category analysed [1].

Performance times were well maintained between 50 and 75 with less than 2% decline in speed per year across all distances. At around 75 years old, performance times declined dramatically by 8% per year suggesting that if disuse were eliminated as a variable function, performance as measured by speed is maintained far past common norms. Evidence of sustained performance with aging is also seen in swimming, cycling, triathlon and weightlifting.

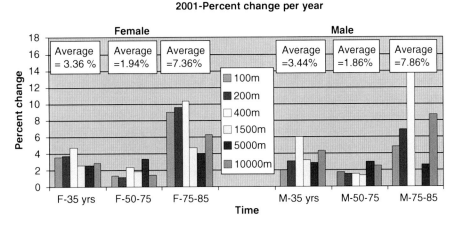

Fig. 1.1 Change in performance with age for Senior Olympians

Chronic Mobility Preserves Lean Muscle Mass

In addition to performance, chronic exercise contributes to the maintenance of lean muscle mass with age. One of the biggest complaints with aging and contributors to frailty is feelings of weakness and objective muscle loss. In population studies, in which up to 60% of participants were sedentary, Walter Frontera and his colleagues found muscle area declines of up to 15% per decade after 50 resulting in significant functional disability. The Health ABC observation of a cohort of 70–79-year-old participants found lean muscle mass replaced with significant volumes of intramuscular adipose tissue and loss of strength.

With chronic exercise these losses of lean muscle mass and strength seem to be prevented. The Performance and Research Initiative for Masters Athletes at the University of Pittsburgh studied masters athletes aged 40–80 who exercised vigorously 4–5 times per week (Fig. 1.2). Lean muscle mass was preserved with minimal intramuscular infiltration of adipose tissue and loss of strength between 40 and 60 with minimal statistically significant decline in age groups after 60 [2].

40-year-old triathlete

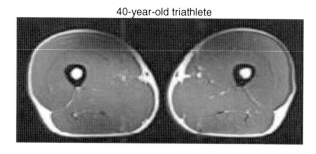

74-year-old sedentary man

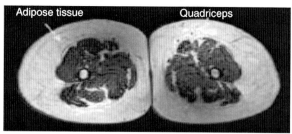

70-year-old triathlete

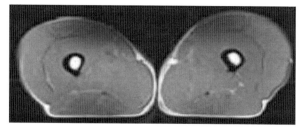

Fig. 1.2 Chronic exercise preserves lean muscle mass in masters athletes

Chronic Impact Sport Predicts Bone Density

Loss of bone density or osteopenia is commonly associated with frailty and fracture in women as they age; however, osteoporosis in men is also a significant problem with more than two million men diagnosed with osteoporosis annually. This loss of bone density results in frailty and fracture that is uniformly disabling but often deadly in elderly men.

Two studies of chronically mobile masters athletes revealed that bone density is preserved in masters athletes when compared to sedentary population. Bone density screenings of masters athletes competing in the Senior Olympics found the prevalence of normal bone density higher in all age groups including the most elderly [1].

A second study [3] found that not only is bone density preserved with chronic exercise, but participation in high-impact sports was a significant predictor of bone mineral density with high-impact exercise contributing as significantly as age, minority status, biologic gender, medication and weight.

Executive Brain Function Maintained in Masters Athletes

Exercise and mobility are known to decrease the symptoms of depression, anxiety, alter brain chemistry, feelings of self-worth and well being and maintain or augment the physical size and function of brain tissue such as the hippocampus. These protective neurocognitive effects are thought to be derived via increased levels of brain derived neurotrophic factor and neurogenesis and are linked to attenuation of age-related mental decline and preservation of mental capacity in physically active people. To evaluate the role of chronic exercise in maintaining executive cognitive function is masters athletes, the University of Pittsburgh's Performance and Research initiative for Masters Athletes studied whether masters athletes, a highly active population, had better cognitive function than age matched controls using the ImPACT neurocognitive assessment tool. Fifty-one pairs of athletes and non-athletes were analyzed and the masters athletes had significantly higher verbal memory scores and faster reaction times than the sedentary controls and scored significantly higher on the physical components of the SF-12. This study begins to detail the preserving effects of exercise and chronic mobility executive cognitive function and highlights the importance of musculoskeletal clinicians in assisting patients to maintain cognitive function via chronic mobility.

The New Science of Aging

Over the last decade, a significant body of research has been generated exploring the age-preserving effects of mobility on the body. Chronic exercise and mobility in masters age athletes maintain performance, bone density, lean muscle mass and even executive brain function. The question is how.

Klothos is a powerful protein, dubbed the longevity protein, that circulates in the extracellular domain and has been associated with lean muscle mass, function and strength, bone density, cardiovascular disease and multiple other age-related diseases. Recent studies found increased Klothos expression with acute exercise in mice and humans with circulating levels associated with increased muscle contraction.

To evaluate whether the same increase in fitness level-related Klothos expression was evident in masters athletes, the PRIMA group performed a pilot study of serum Klothos levels in chronically active masters athletes with those of sedentary controls.

The longevity protein was found in the serum of all masters athletes with levels highest in athletes 50–75 years old compared to athletes over 75 years old. Significantly, all masters athletes, even those over 75 years old expressed higher levels of Klothos than sedentary people younger than 75 years old (unpublished data).

Masterful Care of the Aging Athlete

Data clearly point towards the ability of active people to modify their aging process and change health status via mobility. Performance, lean muscle mass, bone density, cognitive function and multiple metabolic pathways are influenced by mobility, and the work of orthopaedic surgeons and musculoskeletal clinicians is to restore and maintain mobility in our patients via innovative conservative and surgical techniques.

References

1. Wright V, Perricelli B. Age-related rates of performance decline in performance among elite senior athletes. Am J Sports Med. 2008;36:443–50.
2. Wroblewski A, Amati F, Smiley M, Goodpaster B, Wright V. Chronic exercise preserves lean muscle mass in masters athletes. Phys Sportsmed. 2011;39(3):172–8.
3. Leigey D, Irrgang J, Francis K, Cohen P, Wright V. Participation in high-impact sports predicts bone mineral density in senior olympic athletes. Sports Health. 2009;1(6):508–13.

Chapter 2
The New Science of Musculoskeletal Aging in Bone, Muscle, and Tendon/Ligament

Vonda J. Wright and Farah Tejpar

Introduction

As the body ages, changes are seen throughout the musculoskeletal system, namely, within bone, muscle, tendons, and ligaments. An age-related decrease in bone mineral density (BMD), or primary osteoporosis, is defined by the World Health Organization as having a hip or spine BMD of at least 2.5 standard deviations below the mean of young, healthy women measured on dual X-ray absorptiometry. Sarcopenia, or age-related muscle loss, begins at approximately 40 years of age and is more prevalent in the sedentary population. Intrinsic and extrinsic factors associated with aging affect tendon and ligament strength, thus leading to more injuries and prolonged healing time. These changes in the musculoskeletal system can lead to significant disability, thus increasing healthcare costs. Prevention is focused on adequate nutrition, supplements, physical activity, and strength training.

Changes in Bone: Osteoporosis

Osteoporosis is described as low bone mass and changes in the bony architecture that results in bone fragility and increased susceptibility to fracture [1]. It is the most common bone disease in humans [2]. Beginning at 40 years of age, women and men lose approximately 0.5% of their bone mass each year [3]. An estimated 9.9 million

V. J. Wright, MD, MS (✉)
Department of Orthopaedic Surgery, University of Pittsburgh,
UPMC Lemieux Sports Complex, Pittsburgh, PA, USA
e-mail: vonda.wright@northside.com

F. Tejpar, MD
Cleveland Clinic, Weston, FL, USA

© Springer International Publishing AG, part of Springer Nature 2018   9
V. J. Wright, K. K. Middleton (eds.), *Masterful Care of the Aging Athlete*,
https://doi.org/10.1007/978-3-319-16223-2_2

Americans have osteoporosis and 43.1 million have osteopenia or low bone mineral density (BMD). Two million fractures can be attributed to osteoporosis and result in a significant amount of healthcare spending, with 432,000 hospital admissions and over two million physician office visits yearly [2].

There are two classifications for osteoporosis: primary and secondary. Primary osteoporosis is related to the decreased gonadal function with aging, whereas secondary osteoporosis is due to changes in bone metabolism from chronic disease, medications, and nutritional deficiencies [4]. This chapter focuses on primary osteoporosis.

Pathophysiology

Bone is made up of three cell types, osteoblasts, osteoclasts, and osteocytes, and turnover of these cells occurs throughout life [5]. In adults, 90% of the skeleton is comprised of osteocytes, 4–6% is bone-building osteoblasts, and 1–2% is bone-resorbing osteoclasts [4]. During aging, the rate of bone resorbed by osteoclasts is greater than the bone deposited by osteoblasts, thus leading to a loss in bone mass and strength. The change in bone strength is also caused by decreases in cancellous and cortical bone thickness and increases in cortical porosity [6]. Both intrinsic and extrinsic factors affect bone loss. Intrinsic factors include oxidative stress and cellular autophagy. The increased oxidative stress in bone leads to a decrease in the osteoblast lifespan [6]. Extrinsic factors such as sex steroids (e.g., estrogen deficiency), endogenous glucocorticoids, insulin-like growth factor 1 (IGF-1), chronic inflammation, and physical activity lead to increased bone remodeling and resorption. Glucocorticoids inhibit bone formation by stimulating osteoblast apoptosis. With aging, IGF-1, which is important in skeletal growth, can decrease up to 60%. Although the mechanism is unclear, chronic inflammation and decreased physical activity have also been linked to bone loss [6].

Risk Factors, Diagnosis, and Screening

The World Health Organization defines osteoporosis as hip or spine BMD of 2.5 standard deviations or more below the mean of young, healthy women measured on dual X-ray absorptiometry (DXA) [7]. Other techniques such as ultrasound, quantitative computed tomography, and plain radiographs can be used in diagnosis and management of osteoporosis; however, DXA is regarded as the gold standard [8]. The US Preventive Services Task Force (USPSTF) recommends a screening DXA in all women 65 years or older and women 60–64 years with increased fracture risk [9]. The National Osteoporosis Foundation (NOF) recommends a screening DXA in women 65 years or older, men 70 years or older, and any adult with a fracture or risk factors for a fracture [2].

Treatment and Prevention

Oral bisphosphonates, anti-resorptive agents that inhibit osteoclast activity, are the first-line treatment. The two drugs shown to reduce hip and vertebral fractures in men and women are alendronate and risedronate [10, 11]. Prevention of osteoporosis and associated fragility fractures should be focused on maximizing peak bone mass and minimizing bone loss during aging. Animal studies have demonstrated that high-impact weight-bearing activities had beneficial effects on bone density [12]. A study by Leigey et al. conducted with Senior Olympians indicated that high-impact sports contribute positively to BMD in elderly athletes [13]. Additionally, high-impact sports that include balance, leg strength, flexibility, and endurance training were shown to reduce fall risks, thus further preventing fractures [13]. Calcium and vitamin D supplementation in combination with exercise has demonstrated the best results. The recommended requirement of calcium is 1000–1500 mg per day [14]. After 50 years, the requirement increases to 1200–1500 mg per day. Oral vitamin D supplementation of 800–1000 IU per day showed reduced risk of hip and non-vertebral fractures in the elderly. A vitamin D dose of 400 IU per day or less is insufficient to prevent fractures [15]. Additionally, smoking and heavy alcohol intake should be avoided to prevent bone loss.

Changes in Muscle: Sarcopenia

One of the most widely known physiologic changes that occurs with aging is loss of muscle mass. "Sarcopenia" is the age-related decrease in muscle mass, originating from the Greek word "sarcos" meaning flesh and "penia" referring to a lack thereof [16]. It mostly occurs in individuals who lead sedentary lifestyles; however, sarcopenia is also seen in those who are physically active.

Sarcopenia is a major cause of disability and mortality in the elderly and is linked to high healthcare costs in the United States [17]. Approximately 45% of the US population is sarcopenic and 20% have related functional disability. This disability is associated with an increased risk of hospitalization, nursing home placement, and home healthcare. In 2000, an estimated $18.5 billion was spent on sarcopenia-related disability in the United States. Just a 10% reduction in sarcopenia could result in over one billion dollars in savings [17].

Pathophysiology

Skeletal muscle mass gradually decreases from approximately 40 years of age with the greatest loss occurring after age 70 [18]. Men appears to sustain a greater loss of muscle mass compared to women, yet women begin to experience losses at an earlier age compared to men [19]. Studies have shown a 0.47% muscle loss per year in men versus 0.37% muscle loss per year in women. This increases to 0.64–0.70% per year in women and 0.80–0.98% per year in men after age 75. This loss in mass is associated with a loss of strength, with loss of strength occurring 2–5 times more rapidly than loss of mass [16].

In addition to changes in muscle mass, there are changes in muscle fiber distribution that occur with aging. Muscle is composed of type I and II fibers. Type I fibers are small, slow-contracting, low-tension fibers with many mitochondria. Type II fibers are larger, faster-contracting fibers that produce large tension but are quick to fatigue. With aging there is an increase in type I fibers compared to type II fibers [20]. The underlying cause of fiber loss is related to denervation atrophy of single muscle fibers as well as the loss of entire muscle fiber units [20, 21].

Effects of Hormones

Sex hormones play an important role in muscle loss in aging. Circulating testosterone concentrations decrease by 1–3% per year starting at age 35–40 years in men. Approximately 20% of men over age 60 have serum testosterone levels below the normal range. Testosterone deficiency in men not only results in loss of muscle strength and mass but also decreases in bone mass and increases in central body fat. In women, testosterone levels begin to decrease in the fourth decade of life with up to a 50% reduction at the time of menopause [19]. Some of the negative effects of declines in androgens can be reversed with hormone replacement therapy, but the related risks are high. Adverse effects of hormone replacement include prostate cancer, erythrocytosis, and cardiovascular events in men and cancer and venous thromboembolism in women [21].

Diagnostic Imaging

The use of imaging allows for measurement of muscle composition and loss over time. Multiple modalities can be used including DXA, computed tomography (CT), magnetic resonance imaging (MRI), and ultrasonography. DXA) is the most widely used technique due to its availability, low cost, and low exposure to radiation [22, 23]. Computed tomography and MRI provide similar results. The major limitation for CT is the radiation exposure and the limitation for MRI is its cost. Ultrasound is found to be highly reliable in measuring cross-sectional areas of large human muscles. It is good option due to its portability, low cost, and lack of radiation [22].

Treatment and Prevention

Interventions used to prevent and reduce sarcopenia include proper nutrition, increased physical activity, and increased resistance training. Initial treatment of sarcopenia should include an evaluation of protein intake. One study showed that eating half of the recommended dietary intake (RDI) of protein over a 9-week period led to significant reductions in lean body mass in elderly women, whereas those who consumed the recommended intake maintained their lean body mass [24]. Research on masters athletes shows a decline in muscle loss related to high fitness levels and resistance training [18]. It has been documented that older people who engage in regular physical activity and strength training have larger muscles compared to the sedentary population [17]. Fiatarone et al. showed a 9% increase in muscle size after 8 weeks of a high-intensity weight-training program. They also showed a three- to fourfold increase in strength over this period of time [25]. Frontera et al. showed increased strength in the knee flexors and extensors after completion of a 12-week training program in healthy men aged 60–72 years [26]. The American College of Sports Medicine states that resistance training should be an integral part of fitness in older adults, recommending that 1 set of 10–15 repetitions for each major muscle group be performed three times per week [27].

Changes in Tendons and Ligaments

Tendons are regularly arranged collagen fibers that connect muscle to bone [28, 29]. Their main function is to transfer the pull of muscle contraction to the bone [30]. They receive their vascular supply from the musculotendinous junction, the osseo-tendinous junction, and the surrounding vessels. Healthy tendons rely on a normal vascular supply to maintain homeostasis and healing.

Vascular changes play a role in age-related tendinopathy, particularly affecting the rotator cuff, lateral epicondyle forearm extensor, Achilles, quadriceps, and patellar tendons [29]. One study showed 40–50% of patients older than 40 years had degeneration in the rotator cuff and forearm extensor tendons [31]. Age-related changes in tensile strength have been linked to tendon degeneration [29], increased degradative enzyme production [32, 33], and decreased estrogen levels [28].

Ligaments are composed of collagen, elastin, and proteoglycans and connect bone to bone thus stabilizing the joint [29]. Ligaments can be intra-articular or extra-articular. Much of the research on the aging ligament is on the intra-articular anterior cruciate ligament (ACL). Hasegawa et al. evaluated age-related changes in cadaveric ACLs. They found that the earliest changes were in collagen fiber orientation and involved mucoid degeneration, with fiber disorientation being the most prevalent finding in aging ligaments [34]. Another study evaluating the femur-ACL-tibia complex among patients of varying ages found that stiffness, load capacity, and the amount of energy absorbed by the ACL decreased significantly with age [35].

References

1. Kanis JA. Diagnosis of osteoporosis and assessment of fracture risk. Lancet. 2002;359:1929–36.
2. National Osteoporosis Foundation. Physician's guide to prevention and treatment of osteoporosis. http://www.nof.org/professionals/Clinicians_Guide.htm. 1 Apr 2014.
3. Kohrt WM, Bloomfield SA, Little KD, Nelson ME, Yingling VR, American College of Sports Medicine. American College of Sports Medicine Position Stand: physical activity and bone health. Med Sci Sports Exerc. 2004;36(11):1985–96.
4. Syed F, Hoey K. Integrative physiology of the aging bone: insights from animal and cellular models. Ann N Y Acad Sci. 2010:95–106.
5. Carrington JL. Aging bone and cartilage: cross-cutting issues. Biochem Biophys Res Commun. 2005;328:700–8.
6. Almeida M, O'Brien C. Basic biology of skeletal aging: role of stress response pathways. J Gerontol A Biol Sci Med Sci. 2013;68:1197–208.
7. Prevention and management of osteoporosis: report of a WHO Scientific Group. Geneva, Switzerland; 2003. http://whqlibdoc.who.int/trs/WHO_TRS_921.pdf. Accessed 7 Dec 2008.
8. Kanis JA, Gluer CC, for the Committee of Scientific Advisors, International Osteoporosis Foundation. An update on the diagnosis and assessment of osteoporosis with densitometry. Osteoporos Int. 2000;11:192–202.
9. U.S. Department of Health and Human Services. Bone health and osteoporosis: a report of the surgeon general (2004). http://www.surgeongeneral.gov/library/bonehealth/content.html. Accessed 7 Dec 2008.
10. Marcus R, Wong M, Heath H III, Stock JL. Antiresorptive treatment of postmenopausal osteoporosis: comparison of study designs and outcomes in large clinical trials with fracture as an endpoint. Endocr Rev. 2002;23(1):16–37.
11. MacLean C, Newberry S, Maglione M, et al. Systematic review: comparative effectiveness of treatments to prevent fractures in men and women with low bone density or osteoporosis. Ann Intern Med. 2008;148(3):197–213.
12. Turner CH, Robling AG. Designing exercise regimens to increase bone strength. Exerc Sport Sci Rev. 2003;31:45–50.
13. Leigey D, Irrgang J, Francis K, et al. Participation in high-impact sports predicts bone mineral density in senior olympic athletes. Sports Health. 2009;1:508–13.
14. NIH Consensus Conference: Optimal calcium intake: NIH consensus development panel on optimal calcium intake. JAMA. 1994;272:1942–1948.
15. Bischoff-Ferari HA, Willett WC, Wong JB, et al. Fracture prevention with vitamin D supplementation: a meta-analysis of randomized controlled trials. JAMA. 2005;293:2257–64.
16. Mitchell WK, Williams J, Atherton P, et al. Sarcopenia, dynapenia, and the impact of advancing age on the human skeletal muscle size and strength; a quantitative review. Front Physiol. 2012;3:260.
17. Janssen I, Shepard DS, Katzmarzyk PT, et al. The health care cost of sarcopenia in the United States. J Gerontol. 2004;52:80–5.
18. Faulkner JA, Larkin LM, Claflin DR, et al. Age-related changes in the structure and function of skeletal muscles. Clin Exp Pharmacol Physiol. 2007;34:1091–6.
19. Horstman AM, Dillon EL, Urban RJ, et al. The role of androgens and estrogens on healthy aging and longevity. J Gerontol. 2012;67:1140–52.
20. Larsson L, Karlsson J. Isometric and dynamic endurance as a function of age and skeletal muscle characteristics. Acta Physiol Scand. 1978;104:129–36.
21. Siparsky P, Kirkendall D, Garrett W. Muscle changes in aging: understanding sarcopenia. Sports Health. 2014;6:36–40.
22. Cesari M, Fielding R, Pahor M, et al. Biomarkers of sarcopenia in clinical trials- recommendations from the international working group on sarcopenia. J Cachexia Sarcopenia Muscle. 2012;3:181–90.

23. Goodpaster BH, Parks SW, Harris TB, et al. The loss of skeletal muscle strength, mass, and quality in older adults: the health, aging and body composition study. J Gerontol. 2006;61:1059–64.
24. Castaneda C, Charnley JM, Evans WJ, et al. Elderly women accommodate to a low-protein diet with losses of body cell mass, muscle function, and immune response. Am J Clin Nutr. 1995;62:30–9.
25. Fiatarone MA, Marks EC, Ryan ND, et al. High-intensity strength training in nonagenarians. Effects on skeletal muscle. JAMA. 1990;263:3029–34.
26. Frontera WR, Meredith CN, O'Reilly KP, et al. Strength and conditioning in older men: skeletal muscle hypertrophy and improved function. J Appl Physiol. 1988;64:1038–44.
27. American College of Sports Medicine Position Stand. The recommended quantity and quality of exercise for developing and maintaining cardiorespiratory and muscular fitness, and flexibility in healthy adults. Med Sci Sports Exerc. 1998;30:975–91.
28. Frizziero A, Vittadini F, Gasparre G. Impact of oestrogen deficiency and aging on tendon: concise review. Muscles Ligaments Tendons J. 2014;4:324–8.
29. McCarthy M, Hannafin J. The mature athlete: aging tendon and ligament. Sports Health. 2014;6:41–8.
30. Shwartz Y, Blitz E, Zelzer E. One load to rule them all: mechanical control of the musculoskeletal system in development and aging. Differentiation. 2013;86:104–11.
31. Chard MD, Cawston TE, Riley GP, et al. Rotator cuff degeneration and lateral epicondylitis: a comparative histological study. Ann Rheum Dis. 1994;53:30–4.
32. Fu SC, Chan BP, Wang W, et al. Increased expression of matrix metalloproteinase 1 (MMP1) in 11 patients with patellar tendinosis. Acta Orthop Scand. 2002;73:658–62.
33. Lavagnino M, Arnoczky SP. In vitro alterations in cytoskeletal tensional homeostasis control gene expression in tendon cells. J Orthop Res. 2005;23:1211–8.
34. Hasegawa A, Otsuki S, Pauli C, et al. Anterior cruciate ligament changes in the human knee joint in aging and osteoarthritis. Arthritis Rheum. 2012;64:696–704.
35. Woo SL, Hollis JM, Adams DJ, et al. Tensile properties of the human femur-anterior cruciate ligament-tibia complex. The effects of specimen age and orientation. Am J Sports Med. 1991;19:217–25.

Chapter 3
Structural Brain Benefits of Maintained Fitness

Vonda J. Wright and Emily Zhao

Introduction

Exercise is a powerful tool for healthy aging of the body and the mind. Many scientific studies have shown the positive benefits of exercise on the brain. These benefits include maintenance of brain volume in certain areas dedicated to executive function, which is involved in memory, attention, and performing day-to-day tasks. Keeping up with exercise and staying physically fit into the later years of life may protect against the pitfalls of aging, such as cognitive decline, memory loss, and dementia.

A Few Facts About the Brain

The brain is a wonderfully complex organ whose mechanisms scientists have uncovered much about in the last century (Fig. 3.1). The wealth of information on the human brain is much too detailed to discuss here. For the purposes of this chapter, we will present a simplified description of the brain that will attempt to capture the actual processes at work. The brain anatomically is divided into lobes, which serve their own primary functions as well as work together with other lobes for other functions. For example, the frontal lobe is involved with short-term memory, personality, reward, and attention, whereas the temporal lobe is involved more with

V. J. Wright, MD, MS (✉)
Department of Orthopaedic Surgery, University of Pittsburgh,
UPMC Lemieux Sports Complex, Pittsburgh, PA, USA
e-mail: vonda.wright@northside.com

E. Zhao, MD
Department of Orthopaedic Surgery, University of Pittsburgh, Pittsburgh, PA, USA
e-mail: Zhaoe@upmc.edu

© Springer International Publishing AG, part of Springer Nature 2018   17
V. J. Wright, K. K. Middleton (eds.), *Masterful Care of the Aging Athlete*,
https://doi.org/10.1007/978-3-319-16223-2_3

Fig. 3.1 Diagram of the
brain. File:Gray728.svg
from Wikimedia Commons

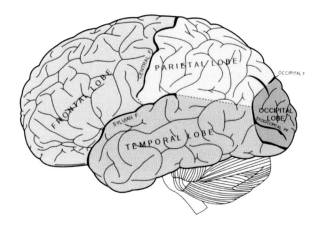

Fig. 3.1 Diagram of the brain. File:Gray728.svg from Wikimedia Commons

language, emotions, and storing memories. The occipital lobe is the brain's primary visual processing area, and the parietal lobe integrates sensory information and also partakes in language processing.

The brain is composed of millions of cells called neurons. Neurons communicate with each other via axons that are insulated by a fatty myelin sheath to allow for faster signaling between cells. The "gray matter" in the brain refers to the neuronal cell bodies, whereas the "white matter" refers to the myelin sheaths. The brain consumes about 20% of the oxygen that we breathe, and 95% of that fuels the gray matter [1].

The area of the brain that we will focus on in this chapter is the temporal lobe, specifically the region known as the hippocampus (Fig. 3.2). The hippocampus is located in the medial temporal lobe on each side of the brain. It serves to consolidate short-term memory into long-term memory and is also involved in spatial navigation, to name a few of its functions. Clinically, this area is significant as it is one of the first areas of the brain to suffer damage in Alzheimer's disease, which is why patients often suffer from memory and orientation problems [2]. It is also the area that scientific studies have demonstrated an association between the size of the hippocampus and exercise, which will be discussed later.

Healthy Versus Unhealthy Brain Aging

From when we are born to early adulthood, our brains grow and make new connections, forming the sophisticated tool that allows us to be who we are and do what we do. As we advance into late adulthood, our brains naturally tend to lose gray matter volume globally, although the loss is not uniform across all parts of the brain. In 1 year, we may lose between 0.2 and 0.5% of our overall brain mass, and depending on the specific region, we may lose up to 3% [2]. In the absence of underlying disease, this process is referred to as "healthy aging" of the brain, and the areas most

Fig. 3.2 The location of
the hippocampus within
the medial temporal lobe

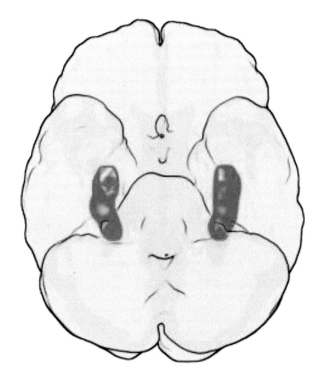

susceptible to age-related decreases in volume are the frontal and temporal lobes. The specific changes in the brain that constitute healthy aging are controversial, as there is much heterogeneity across the population. Research has shown that starting between the ages of 50 and 60 years, we begin to experience a steady decline in mental speed as well as memory formation, possibly related to decreases in temporal lobe volume [3], which includes the hippocampus. Imaging studies have shown that the thickness of the cortices and the gray matter volume in these areas tend to decrease at an accelerated rate in older adults [4], but this is just a process of normal aging of the brain. This process is concerning when it is coupled with clinical evidence of significant cognitive decline which would suggest "unhealthy" aging of the brain.

When we think of unhealthy aging of the brain, we generally think of confusion and memory losses that affect daily life and function. At its onset, these changes are referred to as mild cognitive impairment, and as it worsens, this condition leads to dementia. The biggest risk factor for dementia is age, and one of the consequences of aging, as described previously, is loss of brain volume. Unfortunately, this loss is not predictive of the onset of dementia, as there are other risk factors involved, such as family history, smoking, alcohol abuse, and high blood pressure to name a few. However, one of the hallmarks of dementia is structural changes in the brain. For example, in Alzheimer's dementia, there is global atrophy of gray matter on a much greater scale than what constitutes healthy aging of the brain, along with the characteristic deposition of

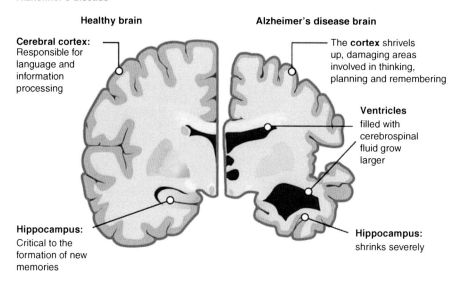

Alzheimer's disease

Healthy brain   **Alzheimer's disease brain**

Cerebral cortex:
Responsible for
language and
information
processing

The **cortex** shrivels
up, damaging areas
involved in thinking,
planning and remembering

Ventricles
filled with
cerebrospinal
fluid grow
larger

Hippocampus:
Critical to the
formation of new
memories

Hippocampus:
shrinks severely

Fig. 3.3 Structural changes in the brain with Alzheimer's disease compared to a healthy brain. Source: Alzheimer's Association

amyloid beta plaques. This atrophy typically begins in the medial temporal lobe structures, including the hippocampus, and expands to include nearby areas such as the medial parietal, lateral temporal, and frontal lobes, eventually spreading to all areas of the brain [5] (Fig. 3.3).

While scientists have not found a cure for dementia—and they certainly have not found a cure for aging – there is a substantial amount of information on how to prevent the negative consequences of aging. The primary focus being to diminish the risk factors (particularly those that are modifiable) that negatively impact healthy aging. This is where exercise comes into play.

Cardiovascular Fitness and Brain Health

Exercise not only has a positive effect on our muscles, but it has a positive effect on our brains as well. There is a wealth of evidence in scientific literature that connects exercise with improved cognitive function [6]. In this literature, the value of exercise is generally measured by self-reported amounts of exercise and through measurements of maximum oxygen capacity during exercise (VO_2 max) Fig. 3.4, which is increased in those with high cardiovascular fitness. Cognitive function is measured both qualitatively and quantitatively through neuropsychological tests that measure memory and problem-solving skills and through neuroimaging such as MRIs.

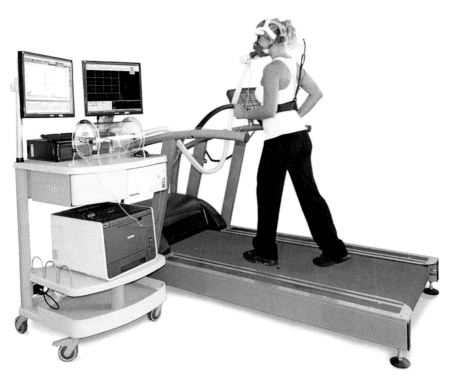

Fig. 3.4 Quantifying cardiorespiratory fitness by measuring VO₂ max. Source: Wikimedia Commons

Studies have shown the positive correlation between higher levels of exercise and higher cognitive abilities. Physically fit older adults perform better at simple cognitive tasks than their less-fit counterparts [7]. A study on 42 women aged 50–90 years showed that higher cardiorespiratory fitness could predict increased overall cognitive function, cognitive speed, verbal memory, and attention [8]. Higher levels of physical activity and increased VO₂ max scores were positively associated with tasks that reflected information processing speed [9]. Increased aerobic capacity with increased age seemed to have the greatest influence on improved cognitive function, especially in areas related to memory and effortful cognitive processing [10]. These results correlate with structural changes seen in the hippocampus and areas mediating executive function. Executive function refers to a set of high-level mental processes that connects past experiences with present actions, such as planning, organizing, paying attention, and problem-solving—of which the hippocampus plays a major role [11]. We are dependent on these executive functions to perform our day-to-day tasks; therefore, it is important to preserve them. These beneficial structural changes in areas of the brain involved in executive function are due to the direct biological impact that exercise has on the brain. Now that we have established that exercise improves fitness, which in turn mediates improved brain function, we shall take a look at the biology behind this process.

The Biology of Exercise in the Brain

Exercise has an immediate biological effect on brain composition and structure. Our brains respond to exercise by producing a protein called brain-derived neurotrophic factor, or BDNF [12]. BDNF is a growth factor, and it functions to preserve survival of existing neurons and to promote the growth of new neurons [13]. It is especially active in the hippocampus, which we described earlier as one of the areas that undergoes age-related decreases in volume. Studies have shown that exercise is associated with decreased loss of hippocampus volume, which is thought to be through the actions of increased BDNF. In essence, exercise helps to slow down hippocampus degeneration, which is one of the first structural signs of aging in the brain. This exercise-induced maintenance of hippocampus size is associated with improved memory function [14].

Multiple studies have shown that participants who engage in 6-month and 1-year aerobic exercise interventions not only had increased fitness but had (1) an increase in serum BDNF levels and measured hippocampus size [14], (2) greater levels of task-related activity in attentional control areas of the brain [15], and (3) greater improvement in short-term memory [16]. One study found that aerobic training for 1 year was associated with hippocampus growth by 2%, which reversed age-related loss by 1–2 years. Also, higher fitness levels in participants prior to beginning a study intervention predicted against age-related hippocampus volume decline [14]. Therefore, age-related loss of brain volume can be slowed down by high levels of lifelong fitness or by starting and maintaining a chronic exercise regimen regardless of prior fitness level. This effect on the brain is mediated by increased levels of BDNF, which is induced by exercise.

In addition to increased hippocampus size and the preservation of gray matter, exercise also helps to preserve white matter mass in the brain. Recall that white matter represents the connections between neurons, and the more learned processes we have, the more white matter we establish. Anterior cortex white matter tract loss is associated with cognitive impairment, dementia, and Alzheimer's disease [17] and is one of the main mechanisms behind cognitive aging. One study found that anterior white matter tracts experienced greater age-related decline than posterior and temporal regions, but this loss was spared by increased aerobic fitness [4]. An area of note is the cingulum, which are white matter tracts that facilitate communication between areas of the limbic system involved in executive function and memory formation. A cross-sectional study of older adults (age 66 ± 6 years) revealed that those with high physical fitness, as measured by VO_2 max, had greater white matter mass in areas of the cingulum compared to older adults who were sedentary [18]. Increased physical activity can help preserve white matter tracts and is one mechanism that may slow down the process of cognitive aging and prevent debilitating mental decline.

Long-Term Fitness and Brain Benefits

The long-term effects of maintained exercise and fitness on the brain are quite evident as well. Various studies have shown that people who report higher levels of exercise over many years are protected against cognitive decline in their later years. Specifically, one study showed that over the span of 8 years, weekly exercise was able to predict higher cognitive function in individuals in their 70s [19]. Another study involving over 300 healthy adults age 55 and over showed that cardiorespiratory fitness, as measured by VO_2 max at the start of the study, was associated with better performance on cognitive function tests after 6 years, compared to their original baseline testing. The strongest associations involved measures of global cognitive function and attention/executive function [20]. This particular study did not re-measure the participants' VO_2 max at the end of the 6-year time period, so we cannot scientifically conclude that their maintained cognitive function was a result of their maintained fitness. However, it is probable that maintaining exercise in these individuals would not have negatively impacted their cognitive scores over time. Even if the participants had stopped exercising or decreased their amounts of exercise, the fitness they had at the start of the study was able to be neuroprotective over a large span of time. It is safe to conclude that chronic exercise and maintained fitness over many years can help prevent neurocognitive decline as well as maintain cognitive processes, well into the golden years of life.

Summary

We all know that exercise is good for our bodies, right now and in the long run. But exercise is also equally good for our minds! Research has shown that exercise can help prevent or slow down age-related decreases in brain volume, especially in the hippocampus region of the temporal lobe, as well as preserve white matter tracts in the anterior region of the brain. This beneficial effect of exercise is protective against cognitive decline and memory loss, so that as we age, our minds can stay just as fit as our bodies.

References

1. Purves D, Augustine GJ, Fitzpatrick D, Hall WC, LaMantia A-S, McNamara JO, et al. Neuroscience. 4th ed. Sunderland: Sinauer Assciates; 2008.
2. Fjell AM, McEvoy L, Holland D, Dale AM, Walhovd KB. What is normal in normal aging? Effects of aging, amyloid and Alzheimer's disease on the cerebral cortex and the hippocampus. Prog Neurobiol. 2014;117:20–40.

3. Nyberg L, Lövdén M, Riklund K, Lindenberger U, Bäckman L. Memory aging and brain maintenance. Trends Cogn Sci. 2012;16(5):292–305.
4. Colcombe SJ, Erickson KI, Raz N, Webb AG, Cohen NJ, McAuley E, et al. Aerobic fitness reduces brain tissue loss in aging humans. J Gerontol A Biol Sci Med Sci. 2003;58(2):176–80.
5. McDonald CR, McEvoy LK, Gharapetian L, Fennema-Notestine C, Hagler DJ Jr, Holland D, et al. Regional rates of neocortical atrophy from normal aging to early Alzheimer disease. Neurology. 2009;73(6):457–65.
6. Zhao E, Tranovich MJ, Wright VJ. The role of mobility as a protective factor of cognitive functioning in aging adults: a review. Sports Health. 2014;6(1):63–9.
7. Colcombe S, Kramer A, McAuley E, Erickson K, Scalf P. Neurocognitive aging and cardiovascular fitness. J Mol Neurosci. 2004;24(1):9–14.
8. Brown AD, McMorris CA, Longman RS, Leigh R, Hill MD, Friedenreich CM, et al. Effects of cardiorespiratory fitness and cerebral blood flow on cognitive outcomes in older women. Neurobiol Aging. 2010;31(12):2047–57.
9. Bixby W, Spalding T, Haufler A, Deeny S, Mahlow P, Zimmerman J, et al. The unique relation of physical activity to executive function in older men and women. Med Sci Sports Exerc. 2007;39(8):1408–16.
10. van Boxtel MP, Paas FG, Houx PJ, Adam JJ, Teeken JC, Jolles J. Aerobic capacity and cognitive performance in a cross-sectional aging study. Med Sci Sports Exerc. 1997;29(10):1357–65.
11. Gilbert SJ, Burgess PW. Executive function. Curr Biol. 2008;18(3):R110–R4.
12. Vaynman S, Ying Z, Gomez-Pinilla F. Hippocampal BDNF mediates the efficacy of exercise on synaptic plasticity and cognition. Eur J Neurosci. 2004;20(10):2580–90.
13. Huang EJ, Reichardt LF. NEUROTROPHINS: roles in neuronal development and function. Annu Rev Neurosci. 2001;24(1):677–736. PubMed PMID: 11520916
14. Erickson KI, Voss MW, Prakash RS, Basak C, Szabo A, Chaddock L, et al. Exercise training increases size of hippocampus and improves memory. Proc Natl Acad Sci. 2011;108(7):3017–22.
15. Colcombe SJ, Kramer AF, Erickson KI, Scalf P, McAuley E, Cohen NJ, et al. Cardiovascular fitness, cortical plasticity, and aging. Proc Natl Acad Sci U S A. 2004;101(9):3316–21.
16. Voss MW, Heo S, Prakash RS, Erickson KI, Alves H, Chaddock L, et al. The influence of aerobic fitness on cerebral white matter integrity and cognitive function in older adults: results of a one-year exercise intervention. Hum Brain Mapp. 2013;34(11):2972–85.
17. Bartzokis G. Age-related myelin breakdown: a developmental model of cognitive decline and Alzheimer's disease. Neurobiol Aging. 2004;25(1):5–18.
18. Marks B, Katz L, Styner M, Smith J. Aerobic fitness and obesity: relationship to cerebral white matter integrity in the brain of active and sedentary older adults. Br J Sports Med. 2011;45(15):1208–15.
19. Weuve J, Kang J, Manson JE, Breteler MB, Ware JH, Grodstein F. Physical activity, including walking, and cognitive function in older women. JAMA. 2004;292(12):1454–61.
20. Barnes DE, Yaffe K, Satariano WA, Tager IB. A longitudinal study of cardiorespiratory fitness and cognitive function in healthy older adults. J Am Geriatr Soc. 2003;51(4):459–65.

Chapter 4
Psychological and/or Mental Health Benefits of Maintaining Activity and Exercise

Vonda J. Wright and Emily Zhao

What Is Mental Health?

Mental health does not just refer to preserving cognitive abilities. The World Health Organization (WHO) defines mental health as "a state of well-being in which every individual realizes his or her own potential, can cope with the normal stresses of life, can work productively and fruitfully, and is able to make a contribution to her or his community" [1]. The WHO definition tells us that the brain is more than just a thought-processing tool; it allows us to have feelings, emotions, desires, motivations, and character. It allows us to function as individuals, be with loved ones in a family, take on jobs, and interact socially with our community. The ability for one to maintain mental health differs among individuals, whether due to family history, upbringing, personal sets of moral values, etc., but just as in cognitive decline, there are ways to try preventing mental health decline. Research has shown that lifelong exercise may be able to contribute toward lifelong mental health.

Mental health disorders are very common in our society. According to the National Comorbidity Survey Replication (NCS-R), a national household survey of the prevalence of mental disorders in the USA [2], about half of Americans will meet the criteria for a mental health disorder sometime in their life. The survey determined that the lifetime prevalence for anxiety disorders was 28.8%, mood disorders (which includes depression) was 20.8%, impulse-control disorders was 24.8%, and substance abuse disorders was 14.6% [3]. While the study showed that some of these disorders have onset of symptoms during adolescence and early

V. J. Wright, MD, MS (✉)
Department of Orthopaedic Surgery,
University of Pittsburgh, UPMC Lemieux Sports Complex, Pittsburgh, PA, USA
e-mail: vonda.wright@northside.com

E. Zhao, MD
Department of Orthopaedic Surgery, University of Pittsburgh, Pittsburgh, PA, USA
e-mail: Zhaoe@upmc.edu

© Springer International Publishing AG, part of Springer Nature 2018   25
V. J. Wright, K. K. Middleton (eds.), *Masterful Care of the Aging Athlete*,
https://doi.org/10.1007/978-3-319-16223-2_4

adulthood, many of these disorders have onset during adulthood at any stage and can be triggered by many environmental factors that may be preventable. Depression and anxiety are two of the most common conditions that affect mental health within the population, and they are also less likely to have genetic and biological roots, as opposed to other disorders such as bipolar disorder and schizophrenia. In this chapter, we will look at how lifelong exercise may be helpful toward maintaining mental health, especially in battling these two diseases.

The Effect of Physical Activity on Depression

Based on the neurobiological model of depression, there is dysregulation of various key biological amines or neurotransmitters within the central nervous system: norepinephrine (NE), dopamine (DA), and serotonin (5-HT). Upregulating these amines are the main targets of pharmacologic treatments for depression. Physical activity and exercise can also have the same antidepressant effects by acting through upregulation via those same biological mechanisms. Various animal and human studies have shown increased metabolites of NE and 5-HT in plasma and urine samples after exercise; however, this result has been difficult to reproduce and confirm widely. In some animal studies, chronic wheel running has been associated with elevated NE levels in the brain. Other studies in animals have found an increase or no change in brain 5-HT levels after acute exercise but an overall decreased turnover of 5-HT with chronic exercise [4]. These studies lack uniformity in experimental methods and data analysis, especially considering the measurement of brain amine levels is usually derived from some other measurement. Other studies have implicated the role of opioid receptors as a mechanism for exercise's effect on mood [5]. Effects mediated by the endogenous opioid system following exercise, such as joy and euphoria, have been able to be reversed by use of naloxone [6]. Despite the complexity involved in understanding the neurobiology of exercise on the brain, the general hypothesis for the role of exercise in the CNS is that exercise stimulates multiple systems that may produce significant short- and long-term antidepressant effects.

Research has supported the implementation of this hypothesis in the clinical treatment of depression. A randomized controlled trial of 202 adults with clinically diagnosed depression who were assigned to 4 months of placebo, pharmacotherapy, home-based exercise therapy, and supervised group exercise therapy showed that the rates of remission tended to be higher for active treatments compared to placebo (supervised exercise = 45%, home-based exercise = 40%, medication = 47%, placebo = 31% ($p = 0.057$)) [7]. The rates of remission showed that exercise treatments were comparable to pharmacotherapy and may be a more advisable when beginning treatment for depression. Another randomized controlled study tried to quantify the dose of exercise that could be responsible for an effect on depression. They found that after 12 weeks, the "public health dose" of 17.5 kcal/kg/week (or about 1500 calories per week for a 200 lb. person) divided into 5 days per week had a higher reduction in the 17-item Hamilton Rating Scale for Depression scores (47%) compared to lower-dose exercise (30%), which was 7 kcal/kg/week divided into three times a week, and placebo (29%) [8]. Before this study was published, there had been no studies that examined the effect of varying frequency, intensity, and duration of exercise on depression. What this study demonstrates is the correlation between higher total energy expenditure and greater reduction in depressive symptoms, which could have important clinical value in treating depression.

The Effect of Physical Activity on Anxiety

Although the neurobiological model of anxiety differs from that of depression, they influence the same pharmacologic targets (DA, NE, and 5-HT), and exercise may facilitate the same beneficial effects on the CNS toward treating anxiety [9]. The amount of research that has been conducted using exercise as a treatment method for anxiety is not as abundant as the research supporting exercises in the treatment of depression. Nonetheless, the available literature does suggest a positive and useful role for exercise in this arena. One study showed that in a group of participants who underwent 8 weeks of aerobic training involving either jogging or walking, those participants who had higher levels of fitness at 6-month follow-up had overall decreased anxiety symptoms compared to baseline [10]. A randomized controlled trial looking at the effects of exercise training in combination with cognitive behavioral therapy saw differing effects of exercise when attempting to treat various anxiety disorders, such as generalized anxiety disorder, social phobia, and agoraphobia [11]. All groups in this study experienced significant reductions in anxiety, depression, and stress scores; however there was a significantly greater reduction in the exercise and CBT groups compared to the control group, confirming the added benefit of exercise therapy in decreasing anxiety.

Long-Term Effects of Maintained Exercise and Fitness on Mental Health

There is much evidence that links long-term exercise to preserved mental health. Cross-sectional surveys examining multiple groups of people in the USA and Canada over the span of 10 years showed that higher levels of physical activity were positively associated with general well-being, lower levels of anxiety and depression, and overall positive mood, and this trend was especially strong in women and people aged 40 and above [12]. Adults randomized to a 12-week aerobic fitness program demonstrated increased fitness as measured by bicycle ergometer test as well as improvement in depression, anxiety, mood, and self-concept scores compared to a control group immediately after fitness intervention, and the improvement in psychological scores for the exercise group were maintained at 1-year follow-up [13].

Similarly, another group of healthy adults who were assigned to a 6-month aerobic fitness program saw improvements in psychological scores related to physical appearance and fitness compared to the control group [14]. These findings suggest that improvements in self-perception could permeate into improvements in other areas of self-worth and well-being, thereby reducing the likelihood of depression and anxiety.

Conclusions

Depression and anxiety are two of the most common debilitating mental health conditions. Fortunately, studies have demonstrated that physical activity and exercise can help treat and even prevent these two conditions. Of course, there are many factors that contribute to mental health, such as comorbid disease, genetics, family history, and social environment. In these cases and other circumstances, exercise may not be as powerful a tool in treating depression and anxiety. However, it is important to note the positive correlation between higher levels of exercise and long-term states of well-being reinforcing the link between a healthy body and a healthy mind. As musculoskeletal clinicians it is important to understand that our roles in maintaining or returning mobility in the lives of our patients can have a profound impact on not only their physical health but in modulating the outcomes of mental health as well.

References

1. Mental health—a state of well-being: World Health Organization; August 2014 [October 23, 2014]. http://www.who.int/features/factfiles/mental_health/en/.
2. Kessler RC, Merikangas KR. The National Comorbidity Survey Replication (NCS-R): background and aims. Int J Methods Psychiatr Res. 2004;13(2):60–8.
3. Kessler RC, Berglund P, Demler O, Jin R, Merikangas KR, Walters EE. LIfetime prevalence and age-of-onset distributions of dsm-iv disorders in the national comorbidity survey replication. Arch Gen Psychiatry. 2005;62(6):593–602.
4. Dunn A, Dishman R. Exercise and the neurobiology of depression. Exerc Sport Sci Rev. 1991;19:41–98.
5. Moore M. Endorphins and exercise: a puzzling relationship. Phys Sportsmed. 1982;10(2):111–4.
6. Janal MN, Colt EWD, Clark WC, Glusman M. Pain sensitivity, mood and plasma endocrine levels in man following long-distance running: Effects of naloxone. Pain. 1984;19(1):13–25.
7. Blumenfeld J, Babyak M, Doraiswamy P. Exercise and pharmacotherapy in the treatment of major depressive disorder. Psychosom Med. 2007;69(7):587–96.
8. Dunn AL, Trivedi MH, Kampert JB, Clark CG, Chambliss HO. Exercise treatment for depression: efficacy and dose response. Am J Prev Med. 2005;28(1):1–8.
9. Anderson E, Shivakumar G. Effects of exercise and physical activity on anxiety. Front Psych. 2013;4(27); Epub Apr 23, 2013.
10. Sexton H, Mære Å, Dahl NH. Exercise intensity and reduction in neurotic symptoms. Acta Psychiatr Scand. 1989;80(3):231–5.

11. Merom D, Phongsavan P, Wagner R, Chey T, Marnane C, Steel Z, et al. Promoting walking as an adjunct intervention to group cognitive behavioral therapy for anxiety disorders—a pilot group randomized trial. J Anxiety Disord. 2008;22(6):959–68.
12. Stephens T. Physical activity and mental health in the United States and Canada: evidence from four population surveys. Prev Med. 1988;17(1):35–47.
13. DiLorenzo TM, Bargman EP, Stucky-Ropp R, Brassington GS, Frensch PA, LaFontaine T. Long-term effects of aerobic exercise on psychological outcomes. Prev Med. 1999;28(1):75–85.
14. King AC, Taylor CB, Haskell WL, DeBusk RF. Influence of regular aerobic exercise on psychological health: a randomized, controlled trial of healthy middle-aged adults. Health Psychol. 1989;8(3):305–24.

Chapter 5
Maximizing Nutrition and Supplements for Masters Athletes

Jeff Lucchino and Kellie K. Middleton

Athletes' Fuel: Eating for Health, Energy, and Longevity

A fundamental component for any athlete's performance is nutrition. Athletes spend months training for one specific event. Often, nutrition is mistakenly left out of their plan, or an afterthought post-event. Nutrition needs to be one of the essential tools in all every athletes' training regimen and toolbox for success. Good nutrition or a healthy "sports diet" can overcome limiting factors that would otherwise cause fatigue or a decrease performance. The fuel demands for many sports are complex and often misunderstood. As such, the goals of this chapter are to review the principles and benefits of healthy nutrition.

What's an effective sports diet? Whether you're at home, traveling for work, or competing, fueling effectively means enjoying at least:

1. Three different food groups at each meal
2. Two different food groups at each snack
3. Evenly sized meals with a reasonable gap of time (3–4 h) throughout the day
4. 90% of calories coming from quality foods and if desired 10% coming from individuals' perceived treat foods

In essence, the key to maximizing a healthy sports diet is to consume a variety of nutrient-dense foods from the five basic food groups. The fundamental components include fruits, vegetables, grains, lean protein, and low-fat dairy. An example of a well-rounded diet from the *MyPlate* guidelines is provided in Table X [1].

J. Lucchino, MS, RD, CSSD, LDN, CPT (✉)
UPMC Lemieux Sports Complex, Pittsburgh, PA, USA
e-mail: lucchinoj@upmc.edu

K. K. Middleton, MD, MPH
Department of Orthopedic Surgery, University of Pittsburgh Medical Center,
Pittsburgh, PA, USA
e-mail: middletonkk@upmc.edu

© Springer International Publishing AG, part of Springer Nature 2018
V. J. Wright, K. K. Middleton (eds.), *Masterful Care of the Aging Athlete*,
https://doi.org/10.1007/978-3-319-16223-2_5

Though generic diet plans incorporating all five fundamental food groups are available, nutrition plans need to be individualized to meet the demands of the individual based on their activity level, body composition, performance goals, food preferences, and responses to various strategies. Appropriate energy intake tailored to meet energy expenditure goals (or energy balance) is vital to assist with training plans geared at manipulating body composition and, in turn, improving musculoskeletal well-being and sports performance.

Micronutrient Breakdown of the Fundamental Five Food Groups

Carbohydrates

Carbohydrates, found in five out of the six categories in the *MyPlate* guidelines, are the foundation of each athlete's sports diet. They comprise a large component of an athlete's dietary intake and receive a great deal of attention for their role in training adaptations. Carbohydrates function as the primary muscle substrate during moderate-high-intensity bouts of activity. By eating carbohydrate-rich fruits, vegetables, grains, and truly any form of starch or sugar (e.g., pasta, potatoes, honey, sports drink, or hard candy), an athlete builds their energy storage in the form of glycogen.

Vegetables and Fruits

Vegetables are excellent fuel sources for athletes. They provide ample vitamins (e.g., vitamin C), minerals (e.g., iron), and hydration. Starchy vegetables such as sweet potatoes, corn, peas, and beets can increase the amount of carbohydrates consumed at a meals. Non-starchy vegetables, particularly salad vegetables, are good sources of fiber, vitamins, and minerals, but they contain a small amount of carbohydrates. If carbohydrate needs are modest, one can add additional non-starchy vegetables into a meal such as a side salad to accompany a pasta dinner.

Fruits are highly variable in their carbohydrate content. Incorporating a variety of fruits as snacks and meals into the sports diet will certainly increase carbohydrate content in a healthy manner. Bananas, apples, and pears to name a few are higher carbohydrate choices, whereas blueberries, strawberries, and blackberries have lower-carbohydrate content. Consuming a variety of fruits helps diversify one's carbohydrate portfolio.

Fruit choices, combinations, and preparations are endless! Fruit is easy to transport and enjoyable to consume because of their natural sweetness. Fruit has a natural sugar (fructose) that is found in different amounts depending on the fruit. Though sugar content is important to monitor, one should focus more on carbohydrate content, vitamins, minerals, and hydration benefits found in fruit rather than trying to avoid particular fruits because of their sugar content.

Dairy Products

Milk and yogurt provide a healthy alternative to increase daily carbohydrate content. Unsweetened varieties offer a lower-carbohydrate content and complement both snacks and meals. Sweetened varieties offer a high content of carbohydrates, which is ideal for individuals with greater carbohydrate demands, such as long-distance runners.

Regardless of fat content in specific dairy foods, the amount of calcium and vitamin D remains consistent. Calcium and vitamin D are affected only when the dairy product is strained, which is a process that removes the whey in protein subsequently decreasing both calcium and vitamin D. Those at risk for osteoporosis and fragility fractures should stick with your plain, regular yogurt for the greatest bone benefit.

Grains

Grains are again an excellent source of energy and fuel for athletes. Grains along with fruits and vegetables make up anywhere from 45–65% 50% of the daily caloric intake in an athletes diet. Whole grains offer an array of B vitamins and fiber. "Quick" and "slow" forms of carbohydrates—referring to the glycemic index (GI)—have been the topic of debate among dietitians and nutritionist, particularly as glycemic index impacts many athletes, but the endurance athlete in particular. The glycemic index is determined based on how 50 g (200 calories) of carbohydrate in a food will affect blood sugar levels after an overnight fast. The glycemic index was initially developed to help people with diabetes manage their blood glucose levels. Athletes started to apply the same principals to manage their blood glucose levels throughout the day, pre-, intra-, and post-workout. There are multiple factors that influence a foods glycemic index including where the food was grown, how it was prepared, and whether the food was consumed on an empty stomach to name a few. Furthermore, daily glycemic response can vary by as much as 43% on any given day [2]. Considering glycemic index as it pertains to athlete meal planning and preparation can be helpful; however, the variability associated with its use must be considered.

Strategic High Sugary Food Timing

Foods high in glucose offer a quick alternative to increase carbohydrate consumption when fueling or refueling requirements are very high. There are specific situations in training or during competitive events when whole grain carbohydrates are not ideal. They can cause bloating, gastrointestinal distress, and possible cramping. Sugary foods, those high in glucose, are fast acting and ideal because of their ability to digest quickly providing energy to muscles in a short period of time. High sugary foods such as sports drinks, sports gels, gummy candy, and sugary beverages are among the top most commonly used items for that quick burst of carbohydrate ingestion before, during, or after training.

When weight loss is desired, high sugary foods should be one of the first items to be reduced. This will allow more room in one's diet for high-fiber, higher-quality, and lower-carbohydrate food choices. Apart from times during competition when sugary sports drinks are needed, athletes should drink plenty of water throughout the day as the main beverage for hydration.

Carbohydrates and Performance

Carbohydrates are known as the "rate-limiting fuel," which puts a great deal of focus on how important exogenous sources of carbohydrates are during training [3]. The average 150-pound (68 kg) male has about 1800 calories of carbohydrate stored in the liver, muscles, blood, and body fluids in approximately the distribution shown in Table 5.1.

Carbohydrates stored in the muscle are easily used during exercise. Those found in the liver maintain appropriate circulating glucose levels throughout the body and are responsible for supplying both the brain and muscle. Carbohydrates are the primary source of energy for the brain and central nervous system and a highly valuable substrate during exercise (especially endurance exercises).

Dietary requirements for carbohydrates vary with an athlete's body composition; the duration of training bouts; environmental factors such as altitude, temperature, and humidity; and training schedule. As such, carbohydrate recommendations should be individualized with each athletes training regimen. An example of carbohydrate needs based on exercise intensity level is provided in Table 5.2.

Many highly competitive athletes will experiment training with low glycogen stores to promote a higher degree of fatty acid oxidation. When the body has to break down fat and protein to produce energy, the process is much slower

Table 5.1 Body's distribution of carbohydrates

Muscle glycogen	1400 calories
Liver glycogen	320 calories
Glucose in body fluids, plasma	80 calories
Total	1800 calories

Adapted from Bartlett J, Hawley J, and Mortion J. 2015. Carbohydrate availability and exercise training adaptation: Too much of a good thing?

Table 5.2 Daily carbohydrate needs

Exercise intensity	Carbohydrate targets
Light (low-intensity or skill-based training)	3–5 g/kg/day of athlete's body weight
Moderate (moderate exercise program: 1 h of daily activity)	5–7 g/kg/day
High (endurance exercise: 1–3 h of moderate-high-intensity exercise)	6–10 g/kg/day
Very high (high-endurance activity: 4–5 h of moderate-high-intensity exercise)	8–12 g/kg/day

Adapted from Burke L, Hawley JA, Wong SHS, and Jeukendrup AE. 2011. "Carbohydrates for training and competition." Journal of Sports Science 29(Supp 1): S17–S27.

Table 5.3 Active carbohydrate-fueling strategies

Types of carbohydrate fueling	Timing	Amounts
General fueling up	Preparation for events <90 min	7–12 g/kg per 24 h
Carbohydrate loading	Preparation for events >90 min of sustained/intermittent exercise	36–48 h of 10–12 g/kg body weight per 24 h
Speedy refueling	<8 h recovery between two fuel-demanding sessions	1–1.2 g/kg/h for first 4 h then resume daily needs
Pre-event fueling	Before exercise >60 min	1–4 g/kg consumed 1–4 h before exercise
During brief exercise	<45 min	Not needed
During sustained high-intensity exercise	45–75 min	Small amounts including mouth rinse
During endurance exercise including "stop and start" sports	1–2.5 h	30–60 g/h
During ultra-endurance exercise	>2.5–3 h	Up to 90 g/h

Adapted from Lukaski HC. Vitamin and mineral status: effects on physical performance. Nutrition. 2004: 20 (7–8):632–644

compared to glycogen breakdown (glycogenolysis). The use of protein and fat instead of carbohydrates for energy production also may lower cardiac output, decrease oxygen uptake, and reduce lactate clearance. Training with low glycogen stores does drive metabolic adaptations to burn fat as the primary energy source. Using fat as fuel sparing glycogen should enhance performance, for fatigue sets in when glycogen is depleted [3]. To date, exercising with low glycogen has been the most effective body fat reduction technique in low-moderate-intensity exercise stages. This is based on research studies with average, untrained non-athletes [4].

Optimizing glycogen storage via exercising with poorly fueled muscles highlights the importance on intra-carbohydrate fueling during endurance training. Carbohydrate feedings during exercise further spare liver glycogen, which, in turn, maintains carbohydrate availability for muscle to use as an energy source. Depletion of these stores is associated with fatigue in the form of reduced work rates, impaired concentration, and increased perceived exertion. Suggestions for carbohydrate fueling are provided in Table 5.3.

Pre-exercise Carbohydrate Infusion

Carbohydrate intake from foods and beverages 3–4 h before competition can fine-tune an athlete's competition fuel storage by optimizing muscle glycogen stores, possibly restoring liver glycogen (for morning training after a fast overnight). The body's primary storage for glycogen is the muscles, which contain the majority of glycogen in the body. In situations of glycogen depletion, the body's first and foremost focus is refilling the muscle glycogen before the liver glycogen. Because of this there's no guarantee in a glycogen depleted state that a carbohydrate-rich meal 3–4 h prior to competition will completely restore liver glycogen. A study by Coyle and Coggan showed that a carbohydrate meal consumed 4 h prior to competition resulted in a 42% elevation in muscle glycogen before activity [5].

Current guidelines for a pre-competition meal (see Table 5.3) suggest a carbohydrate intake of at least 1–4 g/kg of body mass at least 60 min before exercise. The timing of the meal, the amount of carbohydrate, and the overall composition of the meal or snack should be familiar to the athlete to reduce the risk of gastrointestinal distress.

Carbohydrate Intake During Competition

The benefits of carbohydrate consumption during endurance training (greater than 90 min in duration) on stamina and performance is well established in nutrition literature [3]. Carbohydrates can offer an advantage over the pre-exercise meal alone if meal timing and amount are executed properly. This can be challenging as both vary depending on the duration and type of activity. In addition to enhancing performance, intra-competition carbohydrate consumption can decrease central nervous system fatigue [5], improve maintenance of carbohydrate oxidation rates [5], muscle glycogen sparing [5], and maintenance of blood glucose concentrations [5]. See Table 5.3 for recommendations for intra-competition carbohydrate consumption.

Post-exercise Carbohydrate Recovery

The amount and type of food and/or fluid consumption should be just as important as any other meal during the day. The type, duration, and intensity of exercise undertaken will dictate carbohydrate requirements for the post-workout snack. Glycogen restoration is one of the main goals of post-exercise recovery. Refueling requires an adequate amount of carbohydrate to meet recovery needs and to facilitate the muscle-damage repair process and reconditioning. Post-exercise carbohydrate consumption is the most important macronutrient of muscle glycogen synthesis [5]. Co-ingestion of protein and/or amino acids does not further replenish muscle glycogen stores; however, post-exercise protein and/or amino acid does aid in muscle protein synthesis. An intake 0.2–0.4 g/kg/h protein combined with 0.8 g/kg/h stimulates insulin release and results in increased muscle glycogen repletion rates [6].

Protein

Like carbohydrates, protein is just as essential to an athlete's diet. Protein is often overused with the assumed belief that the more protein consumed, the more lean mass you will gain. The Recommended Dietary Allowance (RDA) is 0.66 g of protein per kg of body weight per day for adults over 18 years of age [4, 7].

Based on the acceptable macronutrient distribution range (AMDR), protein should account for 10–35% of total calories consumed. Consuming at least 30 g of protein at meals and spreading the remaining protein at snacks will provide enough essential amino acids for muscle protein synthesis [4]. Essential amino acids – including isoleucine, leucine, lysine, threonine, tryptophan, methionine, histidine, valine, phenylalanine, and arginine – can be generated from dietary protein and also from skeletal muscle breakdown. Specifically three of these ten amino acids play an important role in muscle metabolism. Leucine, isoleucine, and valine (also known as the branched-chain amino acids) aid the body in recovery, muscle metabolism, protein synthesis, protein turnover, and regulation of blood sugar.

Protein is not only vital to muscle rebuilding (not building) and repair, but it also aids in the production of red blood cells, enzymes (three main groups: digestive, metabolic, and food; digestive enzymes breakdown various food groups into useable components; metabolic enzymes are the enzymes your body uses in blood, tissue, and organs; food enzymes are found naturally in food and supply the body enzymes to break down those foods as well), and hormones that are essential for everyday functions. Too little protein leads to chronic fatigue, anemia, muscle wasting, and poor healing and recovery. The key is consuming plenty of high-protein foods that contain the full spectrum of amino acids. Animal sources of protein (meat, eggs, poultry, fish, and dairy) offer a complete protein, or protein that includes all the essential amino acids. Plant-based proteins (nuts, beans, seeds, and legumes) have limited amounts of the essential amino acids. Vegetarian athletes have to work that much harder to reach daily protein goals and must utilize various sources in order to ingest all the essential amino acids regularly.

How Much Protein Is Enough?

Type of athlete	Grams of protein per LB of body weight
Recreational	0.5–0.6
Endurance	0.5–0.8
Strength	0.5–0.8
Teenage	0.7–0.9
Athlete building mass	0.6–0.9
Athlete restricting calories	0.9–1.0
Maximum usable amount	0.9–1.0

Adapted from University of Wisconsin-Milwaukee College of Health Sciences-Department of Kinesiology. The Power of Protein. Presented by Susan Kundrat. Retrieved from http://eatright.org/docs/Kundrat%20-%20POWER%20OF%PROTEIN%20KUNDRAT%20FINAL%2014_14.pdf

Fats

It is well documented that exercise endurance and performance reduce with age, partially secondary to decreased drive and motivation as well as reductions in training frequency and volume. Several strategies to prevent excessive muscle loss in aging athletes have been tested [8], one in particular includes high-fat feeding. In a study done in the 1980s, Dr. Stephen Phinney conducted a test on five well-trained cyclists. They were tested following 1 week of a carbohydrate-rich diet (~57% of energy) and again following 28 days of a severely carbohydrate-restricted (<20 g/day) but isoenergetic diet with energy contributions of 85% fat and 15% protein. Despite the negligible intake of carbohydrate, resting muscle glycogen stores were not depleted but rather reduced to ~45% of values seen on the high-carbohydrate phase. Muscle protein was not used as a fuel source, sparing muscle protein and utilizing the remaining glycogen as the fuel source.

At one point in time, dietary fat was considered bad: "Avoid dietary fat at all costs if you want to change your body composition or athletic performance!" There is some truth to this statement; however, not all fat consumption is bad. In fact, consumption of certain types of fats are vital to athlete health and performance.

Dietary fats aid in the absorption of the fat-soluble vitamins (A, D, E, K), provide essential fatty acids (alpha-linolenic acid (ALA), an omega-3 fatty acid, and linoleic (LA), an omega-6 fatty acid), and may reduce the inflammatory response caused by training that can result in enhanced performance. Athletes should be discouraged to consume an overall dietary fat intake below 20%. Twenty to thirty-five percent is a recommended range for a balanced dietary intake that integrates a healthy amount of dietary fat. Thirty grams or 10% or less of total fat intake should come from saturated fats [4, 9]. Saturated fat is found in greasy meats, red meat, butter, cheese, and cream. Saturated fats are associated with high cholesterol, cardiovascular disease, and possibly even cancer.

Trans-fat or hydrogenated oils are commonly found in commercially prepared products such as muffins, chips, cookies, cakes, and deep-fat fry oils. Trans-fats are considered far worse for your health compared to saturated fats and should be avoided at all cost! Trans-fats are not needed for masters athletes and can be even more detrimental for your overall health compared to saturated fats and, therefore, should not be a part of any sports diet.

The "good" fats that should be incorporated in an athlete's diet are poly- and monounsaturated fats. Poly- and monounsaturated fats can be found in fish, avocados, olives, liquid oils, peanuts, seeds (sesame, sunflower, pumpkin), and nuts (almonds, walnuts, and Brazil nuts). Such fats are essential in the fight against inflammation. Fish especially should be consumed two to three times a week, particularly oily fish (mackerel, herring, and salmon) as these types of fish contain important sources of alpha-linolenic acid (omega-3s), which are vital for heart health, circulation, joint health, and fat metabolism. Additionally, athletes may also want to consider taking fish oil after speaking to his or her physician (see supplement section).

With regard to how fats play a role during performance, intramuscular fats stored as triglyceride are large enough to supply around 2000–3000 calories during exercise. Like muscle glycogen, stores of intramuscular triglycerides also deplete during prolonged exercise. As such, many nutritionists recommend a health daily consumption of fats to contribute to the overall balance between energy consumption and expenditure [10].

Micronutrients

Iron

Iron is a fundamental component of oxygen transport and energy production. Athletes who participate in endurance sports are at an increased risk for iron deficiency due to iron losses through exercise-induced mechanisms that go along with endurance exercise (e.g., sweating, exercise-induced inflammation, hemolysis). Premenopausal female athletes are even more susceptible to anemia secondary to monthly losses during menstruation.

Anemia is clinically defined as hemoglobin (Hgb) less than 12 g/dL (women) and less than 13 g/dL (men). The recommended dietary reference intake (DRI) for iron consumption is set at 18 mg/day for women 51 years or younger, 8 mg/day for women older than 51 years, and as little as 8 mg/day for men. Serum ferritin is the primary index of iron stores. The physiological range of serum ferritin in adult women is 15–150 µg/L and 15–200 µg/L for men. Increasing iron dietary intake or supplementation are the only two ways to replace iron losses and replete iron stores. Dietary iron stores come in two forms: heme and non-heme. Heme is present within hemoglobin and myoglobin. The heme form of iron is from animal sources, while the non-heme is found in plant sources. Heme iron uptake can be as efficient as 40%; however heme iron typically constitutes only about 10% of all dietary iron [11–13].

Calcium and Vitamin D

Calcium is extremely important for growth, maintenance, and repair of bone tissue, regulation of muscle contraction, nerve conduction, and normal blood clotting. Low calcium stores predispose athletes to osteopenia, osteoporosis, and, ultimately, fragility fractures. Dietary calcium is optimally absorbed with the assistance of vitamin D. As such, both calcium intake of 1500 mg/day *and* vitamin D (1500–2000 IU/day) are necessary to optimize bone health [13, 15].

It is well recognized that vitamin D is necessary to promote optimal bone health; however, there is also substantial evidence that vitamin D deficiency has a profound negative effect on immunity, inflammation, and muscular function. Adequate daily intakes for vitamin D for adults up to 50 years of age are 200 international units (IU), 400 IU for adults age 51–70, and 600 IU for adults aged 71 years or older. Vitamin D deficiency can indirectly interfere with an athlete's ability to train and perform at a highly competitive level. Those athletes with the highest risk include those with limited sun exposure, those who practice outdoors in the early morning or late afternoon, and/or those athletes with darker skin complexions. Vitamin D is produced in the body in a process that starts when rays in the invisible ultraviolet B (UVB) parts of the light spectrum are absorbed by the skin. Where you live can affect this; higher latitudes have lower levels of vitamin D-producing UVB light that reaches the earth's surface in the winter time because of the low angle of the sun. Darker skin complexions need more sun exposure due to a substance called melanin which is found in higher amounts with people with darker complexions. Melanin competes for UVB with the substance in the skin that produces vitamin D.

With respect to vitamin D stores, it is very important to have both vitamin D and calcium levels assessed. The ideal vitamin D level (in the most active form of 1,25-dihydroxyvitamin D3) is at least 50 nmol/L. To achieve this level, medical professionals and nutritionists recommend safe sun exposure (twice a week between 10 am and 3 pm) and/or dietary supplement with 1000–2000 IU vitamin D3 per day. Vitamin D can also be obtained from the diet; however, natural sources are limited (cod-liver oil, wild salmon, sun-dried shiitake mushrooms, and canned sardines). Fortified sources including fatty fish, fortified milk, margarine, and cereal are becoming more common [11, 13, 23].

Hydration and Fluid Balance Guidelines

Adequate fluid consumption daily, before, and after training helps maintain hydration and optimal performance. Consumption of 17 ounces of fluid 2 h prior to training promotes hydration and allows time for excretion of excess ingested water. Consumption of fluids during activity should be early and often to efficiently replace fluids lost during training. Carbohydrates and/or electrolytes should additionally be consumed for exercise lasting greater than 60 min in duration. Ingestion of 30–60 g of carbohydrates/h (4–8% carbohydrate in the fluid or 13–18 g of carbohydrates per 8 oz) after the first hour is recommended for oxidation of carbo-hydrates and to delay the onset of fatigue. Carbohydrates can be consumed in the form of sugar (e.g., glucose or sucrose) or starch (e.g., maltodextrin). Electrolytes (primarily sodium) reduce the risks of hyponatremia: 0.5–0.7 g of sodium per liter of water is appropriate to replace sweat losses from activities greater than 1 h in length [14, 15].

Dehydration (i.e., 2% body weight loss) can elicit a 20% or greater reduction in cardiac output and over a period of time has the potential for development of heat-related disorders [13]. Even a small degree of dehydration can increase the rate of perceived exertion and limit the body's ability to dissipate heat. This, in turn, can raise the body's internal temperature to dangerous levels predisposing an athlete to life-threating heat stroke. To prevent this from occurring, water losses during exercise should be replaced at a rate comparable to an athlete's sweat rate. If water losses are not completely met during exercise, consumption of 24 oz. of fluid for every pound of weight lost during exercise will assist in complete fluid replacement.

Supplements

Whey Protein

Whey protein is a very common supplement that's been around for decades. Various forms of whey protein (isolate, hydrolysate, concentrate) have recently come onto the market with whey isolate being one of the highest quality forms of whey pro-teins. It has an efficient absorption and digestion rate that is ideal for an increase in muscle protein synthesis (MPS) post-training. Ten to twenty grams of whey protein post-workout has been shown to maximally stimulate MPS [9, 16, 17].

After the age of 30, muscle loss occurs at the rate of 5% per decade. Aging is accompanied by sarcopenia, or a progressive decline in skeletal muscle mass. Furthermore, recent data suggests that skeletal muscle protein metabolism in response to food intake is impaired in older adults. Ingestion of proteins in the form of free amino acids, beef, or milk protein strongly stimulates MPS. Whey protein is more effective than soy, casein, or hydrolyzed casein at promoting postprandial muscle protein accretion and sparing muscle protein during an energy restriction phase [9, 16].

Fish Oil

Oily fish and fish oils contain the long-chain omega-3 fatty acids, eicosapentaenoic acid (EPA), and docosahexaenoic acid (DHA). From several studies, a dose of any-where from 2 to 3 g of fish oil per day may have positive effects on reduction of oxida-tive stress, enhanced stroke volume and cardiac output responses to moderate-intensity exercises, reduction in exercise-induced soreness, and improvements in muscle strength and functional capacity (the extent to which a person can increase exercise intensity levels and maintain those levels) of elderly women [8, 10].

Caffeine

Caffeine may be the most widely used stimulant in the word. The average caffeine consumption in the United States is 200 mg or approximately two cups of coffee per day. Caffeine is often referred to as an ergogenic aid, but it has no nutritional value. Ingested caffeine is quickly absorbed from the stomach and peaks in the blood in 1–2 h time. Research [Harris MH] has shown that ingestion of 3–9 mg of caffeine per kilogram of body weight 1 h prior to exercise increased endurance running and cycling performance in the laboratory [12]. To put this into perspective, a 150 lb (68 kg) endurance athlete's range of caffeine consumption is 204–612 mg of caffeine [12, 18]. The caffeine-containing supplements on the market today vary drastically in the caffeine dosage. Higher dosages (greater than 400 mg) have not yet been proven effective in a clinical setting. Therefore when it comes to caffeine, more has not yet been proven to be better in the health or performance perspective.

References

1. Food Pyramid. ChooseMyPlate.gov - MyPlate Dietary Guidelines.
2. Vega-Lopez S, Ausman LM, Griffith JL, Lichtenstein AH. Inter-individual reproducibility of glycemic index values for commercial white bread. Diabetes Care. 2007;30:1412–7.
3. Bartlett J, Hawley J, Mortion J. Carbohydrate availability and exercise training adaptation: too much of a good thing? Eur J Sport Sci. 2015;15(1):3–12.
4. Dietary reference intakes: macronutrients. Acceptable macronutrient distribution range. Institute of Medicine. 2005;4(4):193–8.
5. Burke L, Hawley JA, Wong SHS, Jeukendrup AE. Carbohydrates for training and competition. J Sports Sci. 2011;29(Supp 1):S17–27.
6. Beelen M, Burke LM, Gibala MJ, van Loon LJ. Nutritional strategies to promote postexercise recovery. Int J Sport Nutr Exerc Metab. 2010;20(6):515–32.
7. United States Department of Agriculture. Dietary Reference Intake (DRIs): Estimated average requirements.
8. Burke L. Re-examining high-fat diets for sports performance. Did we call the 'nail in the coffin' too soon? Sports Med. 2015;45(Supplement 1):33–49.
9. Tipton KD, Rasmussen BB, Miller SL, Wolf SE, Owens-Stovall SK, Petrini BE, Wolfe RR. Timing of amino acid-carbohydrate ingestion alters metabolic response of muscle to resistance exercise. Am J Physiol Endocrinol Metab. 2001;281(2):E197–206.
10. Hawley J. Effect of increased fat availability on metabolism and exercise capacity. Med Sci Sports Exerc. 2002;34(9):1485–91.
11. DellaValle DM. Iron supplementation for female athletes: effects on iron status and performance outcomes. Curr Sports Med Rep. 2013;12(4):234–9.
12. Harris MH. Dietary supplements and sports performance: minerals. J Int Soc Sports Nutr. 2005;2(1):43–9.

13. Lukaski HC. Vitamin and mineral status: effects on physical performance. Nutrition. 2004; 20(7–8):632–44.
14. American College of Sports Medicine. Position stand: exercise and fluid replacement. Med Sci Sports Exerc. 2007;39(2):377–90.
15. Medicine & Science in Sports & Exercise: 2016. Joint Position Statement. 48(3):543–68.
16. Phillips SM. Dietary protein for athletes: from requirements to optimum adaptation. J Sports Sci. 2011;29(Supp 1):S29–38.
17. University of Wisconsin-Milwaukee College of Health Sciences-Department of Kinesiology. The power of protein. Presented by Susan Kundrat. Retrieved from http://eatright.org/docs/ Kundrat%20-%20POWER%20OF%PROTEIN%20KUNDRAT%20FINAL%2014_14.pdf.
18. Tarnopolsky MA. Caffeine and creatine use in sport. Ann Nutr Metab. 2010;57(Suppl 2):1–8.

Chapter 6
Antiaging and Performance-Enhancing Drugs

Zaneb Yaseen

Testosterone

Testosterone (T) supplements have been one of the most widely prescribed medications over the last 10 years [1]. Testosterone is an androgenic steroid hormone that is involved in a variety of physiological functions including sexual function and development [2, 3]. It is predominantly synthesized by the testicular Leydig cells in response to luteinizing hormone. It can activate androgen receptors by directly binding to androgen receptors as well as via conversion into dihydrotestosterone (DHT), which has an even greater affinity for receptors. These all serve to promote sexual development. Interestingly, T can also be converted to estradiol by the aromatase enzyme. Estradiol binds to estrogen receptors and, in turn, acts on bone. Which further illustrates its importance in the maintenance of bone mineral density [2]. Conversion to estradiol also serves to stimulate normal sexual function and libido and erectile function as well as decrease subcutaneous and intra-abdominal body fat in men [4].

Pathophysiology of Low T

Many studies have demonstrated a decline in serum testosterone concentration and free testosterone with aging, but an increase in sex hormone-binding globulin (SHBG) [5–7]. In men, this process is analogous to menopause in women and is often referred to as andropause, androgren deficiency in the aging male, or partial androgen deficiency in the aging male [8]. This decline can begin as early as the

Z. Yaseen, MD
Department of Orthopaedic Surgery, Cayuga Medical Associates, Ithaca, NY, USA
e-mail: zyaseen@cayugamedicalassociates.org

third decade of life with an estimate decrease of 1% each year after age 30 [9]. Low testosterone is defined as serum levels <300 ng/dL.

The full effects and clinical consequences have yet to be fully appreciated, unlike menopause, which is better described. Aside from a decline in sexual function and its association with low testosterone levels, there are other potential associations that relate to aging such as loss of strength and muscle mass and an increase in fat stores, cardiovascular issues, osteoporosis, and anemia. Additionally, decrease testosterone influences mood and cognitive function.

During the aging process, muscle strength and overall power decrease due to loss of muscle mass. Each year healthy adults over the age of 50 lose approximately 1–2% of their skeletal muscle. This process is also known as sarcopenia [10–12]. This muscle loss is also accompanied with an increase in fat stores [13]. Comparison of low testosterone (or hypogonadal) men with eugonadal controls demonstrated a greater percentage body fat in those with low testosterone [14]. Exact mechanisms of muscle loss are likely multifactorial but include malnutrition, physical inactivity or muscle unloading, as well as hypogonadism. Sarcopenia coupled with an increase in fat stores is suspected to affect the cardiovascular system. Specifically, the decreased muscle mass and increased fat stores lead to central obesity, insulin resistance, and a potentially increased mortality.

A study evaluating a population-based cohort of men found that low levels of testosterone, SHBG, and clinical androgen deficiency are associated with an increased risk of developing metabolic syndrome even with a normal BMI [15, 16]. This couples with increasing evidence to suggest that low testosterone levels are associated with coronary artery disease (CAD) [17]. Testosterone levels are known to affect the lipid profile specifically having a positive effect on high-density lipoprotein (HDL) cholesterol and a negative effect on the more atherogenic low-density lipoprotein (LDL), cholesterol, and triglycerides [18, 19].

Other consequences of low testosterone include decrease in bone mineral density (BMD) [20, 21], which leads to an increase fracture risk. A prospective cohort study demonstrated that the risk of non-vertebral fractures in men over 65 years of age was increased in men with low testosterone and estradiol and high SHBG [22]. Low T is also associated with an increase in depressive symptoms or mood changes [23, 24]. Furthermore, a decrease in cognitive function has been observed—specifically, low T has been linked to memory, visuospatial performance, and a faster decline in visual memory [25, 26].

Testosterone Supplementation

Studies on T supplementation have demonstrated improvements in several areas including muscle mass, body fat, cardiovascular profile, bone mineral density, mood, and cognition. Katznelson et al. found that treatment for 18 months of testosterone enanthate in hypogonadal men resulted in an increase in lean muscle mass and a decrease in subcutaneous fat [14]. A meta-analysis of 11 studies examining the relationship between androgen treatment and muscle strength determined a moderate increase in muscle strength in men 65 years and older [27, 28].

Other studies have demonstrated an improvement in lipid profiles of elderly and hypogonadal men including reductions in total and LDL cholesterol with T supplementation [19, 28]. T replacement has also been shown to reduce associated CAD in animal models and improve myocardial ischemia in men with angina pectoris. These studies have suggested that formation and development of atherosclerosis is affected by levels of T and replenishing them is beneficial [17]. Studies examining the effect of intravenous T supplementation have demonstrated incredible medical benefits including improvements in exercise performance via treadmill testing and a reduction in angina [19].

Studies examining BMD of the spine and hip after T administrations have demonstrated beneficial effects whether an increase in BMD or maintenance of BMD [29, 30]. In one of these studies, outcomes were related to the degree of T deficiency, i.e., how low pretreatment T levels were [29]. Katznelson et al. also described improvements in BMD of the spine and trabecular bone [14]. Another study examined higher-dose T with and without finasteride (a 5-alpha-reductase inhibitor that converts T to DHT). In both treatment groups, T levels were elevated to those higher than mid-normal for young men. Such gains were shown to significantly increase spine and hip BMD in both groups [31]. A meta-analysis of placebo-controlled trials demonstrated that, in general, intramuscular administration resulted in a better response than transdermal T supplementation. Additionally, authors found that T treatment resulted in a moderate increase in lumbar BMD with an inconclusive effect on the BMD of the femoral neck [32].

As previously mentioned, low T is also thought to affect mood and cognitive function. T replacement has been found to improve subthreshold depression (dysthymia) [33]. A randomized, multicenter study demonstrated an improvement in positive mood with a significant decline in negative mood in all subjects after 180 days of treatment [34]. Another study trialed T therapy as a treatment for depression in patients with low and low-normal testosterone levels. After 6 weeks of therapy, 54% had improvement in their outcome measures [35]. T supplementation is also associated with enhancements of spatial cognition and improvements in verbal memory. This effect is believed to be mediated through the estradiol pathway [36, 37].

Significant research efforts have demonstrated the benefits of testosterone in males who have low T levels. Interestingly, recent studies have also demonstrated some benefit to T supplementation in women. Supplementation in obese and premenopausal women was found to increase protein synthesis by 45% but did not affect the lipid profile significantly [34]. Though such studies are promising, additional research is needed to further evaluate the role of T supplementation in women's health.

In 2006, the Endocrine Society Practice Guidelines recommended replacing testosterone in order to improve sexual function, sense of well-being, muscle mass and strength, and bone mineral density in men with symptoms of androgen deficiency that had low testosterone levels. These recommendations extend to those patients who also have breast or prostate cancer. T levels should be regularly monitored and restored to a mid-normal range [38].

Complications

All medications and supplements must be utilized cautiously with an understanding of potential side effects and treatment complications. Numerous studies have reported adverse outcomes with testosterone therapy. In a recent JAMA article, Vigen et al. reported results from their retrospective national cohort study of men in the Veterans Affairs system with diagnosed low testosterone that either underwent testosterone therapy or no therapy following coronary angiography. They found that there was a higher risk for an event (death, myocardial infarction, ischemic stroke) in those who underwent testosterone therapy even with lower baseline comorbidities. They noted the association was consistent with or without previous CAD [39]. It is important to note that there were numerous criticisms of the paper, including the methodology.

A review and meta-analysis by Borst et al. found that cardiovascular risks were dependent upon route of administration; oral medications posed the most significant risk. There were no significant cardiovascular effects noted with either injectable or transdermal testosterone [40]. On the contrary, Corona et al. determined that there is no causal role between T therapy and cardiovascular events in their meta-analysis including 75 studies. Furthermore, the authors found that in subjects with metabolic derangements, there was a protective effect of T therapy on cardiovascular risk [28]. Other adverse risks associated with T supplements include polycythemia and an increase in detection of prostate events, but *not* prostate cancer [41]. There are also adverse effects of T supplementation associated with the route of administration such as redness and pain at the injection site. Less reported adverse outcomes include breast tenderness, gynecomastia, and worsening sleep apnea [42].

Resveratrol

Resveratrol (Rsv) is a naturally occurring polyphenol, classified as a phytoalexin, that is found in plants that have undergone environmental stress. Most notably, it is found in grape skins but also in other plants such as raspberries, blueberries, and even peanuts [43, 44]. The most significant dietary source is red wine, which is suspected to be the reason for the French Paradox: the phenomenon that the French population has a 40% lower rate of cardiovascular disease than the rest of Europe even with a diet rich in saturated fat [45, 46].

Treatment

Resveratrol has multiple therapeutic properties including anti-inflammatory, cardio-protective, and even anticancer effects [47, 48]. Numerous in vivo studies have confirmed that administration of Rsv can prevent protein degradation even when exposed to glucocorticoids and tumor necrosis factor (TNF)-alpha [49]. This exerts protective effect on muscle wasting under different stress states such as cachexia and disuse [48]. A recent study in the rat model demonstrated that resveratrol administration alone (in the absence of fluid administration) during resuscitation improved survival following hemorrhagic injury [50].

Several human clinical trials have also shown promising effects from Rsv treatment. A double-blinded, randomized, crossover study in obese patients found that Rsv in the form of dietary grape powder had beneficial effects on lipid profile by decreasing concentrations of large LDL and large LDL-cholesterol particles. They also noted an increase in IL-6 and IL-1β. The authors concluded that the grape powder may decrease atherogenic lipid factors that potentially lead to cardiovascular disease [51]. Other studies also found that grape powder led to beneficial effects such as reduced blood pressure, decreased circulating cell adhesion molecules (CAMs), improvement in plasma lipids, inflammatory cytokines, and oxidative stress [47]. Prior et al. demonstrated that consumption of blueberries, mixed grapes, and kiwifruit were associated with an increase in plasma antioxidant capacity in blood samples [52]. A phase 1 trial examined the effect of Rsv derivatives on colon cancer patients with examination of the effects of *wnt* gene expression in healthy tissue and cancer tissue. Preliminary results demonstrated an inhibition of the *wnt* pathway in normal colonic cells but no effect in the cancer cells. This suggests that this supplement could possibly be used to prevent colon cancer; however, further studies are warranted prior to drawing any firm positive conclusions [53].

Complications

Although grapes and most other fruits are safe and nontoxic, some formulations of grape derivatives have potential side effects. Rsv administration demonstrated cytotoxicity in multiple myeloma (MM) cell lines and inhibited nuclear factor kappa-B, AKT, and signal transducer and activator of transcription 3, which are all genetic factors involved in cancer cell growth cascades. In fact, the combination of Rsv with bortezomib (a proteasome inhibitor used as a chemotherapy drug in the treatment of multiple myeloma and mantle cell lymphoma) achieved synergistic cytotoxicity in vitro [54]. As such, Popat et al. sought to evaluate the combination of Rsv (SRT501) with bortezomib for clinical development. Unfortunately, renal failure was observed in a number of patients. The authors concluded that SRT501 and bortezomib demonstrated an unacceptable safety profile and minimal efficiency in patients with relapsed/refractory multiple myeloma [55].

In conclusion, there are potential benefits to Rsv. However, it is important to realize that although resveratrol has been studied for the last three decades with numerous beneficial effects, these are almost all limited to animal or cell models. Such findings may not translate to the human model [56]. Further research efforts are needed to define and limit adverse affects in humans and to determine the optimal dose needed to express the proposed health benefits.

Growth Hormone

Growth hormone (GH) is produced in the pituitary and acts to stimulate the liver to synthesize insulin-like growth factor 1 (IGF-1). This, in turn, stimulates linear growth in children [57]. It has numerous actions such as increased lipolysis (mobilization of stored triglyceride); stimulation of protein synthesis; antagonism of molecules such as insulin, phosphate, and sodium; and water retention [58]. Secretion is mostly pulsatile and influenced by sleep (slow wave), nutrition, and even physical activity [57, 59, 60].

GH secretion is mediated by somatostatin, growth hormone-releasing hormone, and ghrelin. Somatostatin inhibits GH secretion and the secretion of other hormones as well. Contrarily, growth hormone-releasing hormone (GHRH) stimulates GH release and synthesis [2, 61].

Pathophysiology

Secretion and serum levels of GH decrease with age [57, 61, 62]. It is estimated that this decline is about 15% for each decade of life after the third decade [61]. This is likely due to a decrease in response of the pituitary when subjected to growth hormone-releasing hormone as well as a decrease in the releasing hormone itself [63, 64]. It could also be due to an increase in secretion of somatostatin [61]. This decrease is responsible for a decrease in lean body mass, increased intra-abdominal fat, and thinning of the skin [62, 65], as well as decreased aerobic capacity, affective disturbances, abnormal lipids, and increased vascular mortality [57]. GH deficiency is also associated with a decrease in BMD, bone mineral content, and an increased fracture risk [62]. Changes in cognitive function also occur, along with changes to sleep patterns, particularly slow wave sleep. Age-related decline in GH and other hormones may also be related to a decline in cognition [66].

Treatment

There has been a plethora of research devoted to GH deficiency in animal models, children, adolescents, and nonelderly adults, which has been extrapolated to the adult aging population. A randomized, double-blind, placebo-controlled trial, performed in healthy men and women (aged 65–88), examined the effect of GH and found that administration increased lean body mass and decreased fat mass [58]. Body composition was examined in men over 61 years old who underwent injection of biosynthetic human growth hormone. They noted an increase in lean body mass of 6%, decrease of adipose mass of −15%, as well as a 4% improvement in skin thickness [67].

Another study examined recombinant human GH replacement in adults with GH deficiency for at least 5 years of therapy. They found that in men who were treated for at least 15 years, there was an increase in BMD in the lumbar spine and maintenance of hip BMD [68]. Cognitive studies in rodents suggest that administration of GH could improve cognitive function, vascularity, neurogenesis, and glucose [61, 69]. Studies in the animal model demonstrated improved learning and memory in aging rats as well as decreased cell death [69]. Vitiello et al. studied the effects of GHRH or placebo on patients aged 89 or older for 6 months. They found an improved performance in cognition including picture arrangement, verbal sets, and even IQ [66].

Complications

Despite the overwhelmingly positive effects of GH treatment, some adverse effects have been reported. Blackman et al. noted that in their otherwise healthy subjects, glucose intolerance and diabetes occurred rather frequently. They also noted edema, carpal tunnel syndrome particularly in men, gynecomastia, and arthralgia [58, 67, 70]. Many of these side effects disappeared with 3 months of cessation of treatment. A recent randomized controlled study discussed short- and long-term GH replacement and found no consistent increase in diabetes regardless of length of treatment. They also did not report any increase risk in primary cancer, secondary neoplasia, nor recurrence of previous tumors. However, they did have a small study population [71].

In conclusion, GH treatment does improve lean body mass and reduces fat stores. However, similar to most supplements and hormone replacement therapies, further studies are needed to assess if there are other concrete benefits and to identify detrimental side effects.

Selective Androgen Receptor Modulators

Selective androgen receptor modulators (SARMs) are nonsteroidal molecules that bind selectively to tissues with androgen receptors. The ideal purpose is to cause an anabolic effect on muscle and bone while sparing any activation of the prostate and secondary sex organs [3, 12, 72]. Unlike testosterone, the molecules cannot be converted into active metabolites such as estradiol and dihydrotestosterone (DHT) [73].

Enobosarm (GTx-024, S-22, Ostarine™) is derived from the antiandrogen bicalutamide and belongs to the class of aryl proprionamides. Ostarine™ is currently a phase II study drug designed to combat sarcopenia by selectively increasing muscle performance and mass in elderly men and women. Early studies have demonstrated improvement in ability to climb stairs, increases in lean body mass, and decrease in fat mass. These changes have occurred without affecting prostate-specific antigen levels in male subjects and affecting hair growth in women [3]. Other developing studies focusing on cachexia in the cancer population and enobosarm have demonstrated improvements in lean body mass and function in power. Phase I trials demonstrated improvement in lean body mass, thigh muscle volume, and leg strength after 12 weeks of use in postmenopausal women. Phase II studies demonstrated a dose-dependent increase in lean body mass in males and postmenopausal females over the age of 60 who took the drug for 86 days. They also noted a significant decrease in total fat mass, time needed to climb stairs, as well as an increase in stair climb power. Blood work demonstrated overall decline in blood glucose, plasma insulin levels, and serum triglycerides in the higher-dose group. High-density lipoproteins also declined depending upon dose with no effect on low-density lipoproteins. DHT and estradiol levels did not change. Phase II trials in cancer patients also demonstrated statistically significant increase in total lean body mass, decrease in time to climb stairs, and increase in stair climb power with both low- and high-dose enobosarm arms [10, 74]. A phase III trial has completed enrollment in patients with stage III and IV non-small cell lung cancer with specific aims for prevention and treatment of muscle wasting. Early results have demonstrated a positive effect on lean body mass. Adverse effects most commonly include headache, back pain, fatigue, nausea, diarrhea, and flu-like illness, but overall the drug was well tolerated. Few patients in the phase II trials experienced a transient increase in liver enzymes that resolved with cessation of drug use [10, 75].

Since androgens can affect osteoporosis and overall bone mass, SARMs could be used in both men and women due to its selective effect. Animal studies examining the effect of S-4, an aryl propionamide, on ovariectomized rats demonstrated a multitude of positive effects compared to ovariectomized with other drug or no intervention (DHT) and the intact group with or without drug. The S-4-treated ovariectomized group demonstrated maintenance of bone mass, decrease in fat mass, and maintenance of cortical thickness of bone compared to control and DHT groups. All the S-4-treated groups also demonstrated maintenance of strength of bone with three-point bending analysis. Interestingly, the intact group given S-4 demonstrated an increase of trabecular bone mineral density. Further examination of the bone sparing effects demonstrated an anabolic effect of S-4 [76].

In summary, these drugs may be safe and effective in preventing lean muscle wasting in the aging population as well as the ill population. Preliminary studies in the animal model have demonstrated an overall positive effect on bone mass. Further studies are being developed to determine the full effects of SARMs on humans with regard to increasing lean muscle mass and strength as well as preventing bone loss. Due to its anabolic nature, SARM has been banned by the World Anti-Doping Agency since January 2008.

Mammalian Target of Rapamycin

Mammalian target of rapamycin (mTOR) has been shown to modulate aging in a multitude of organisms from yeasts to small mammals [77, 78]. Rapamycin (also known as sirolimus) is a compound, produced from the bacterium *Streptomyces hygroscopicus*, found on the island of Rapa Nui [77, 78]. Throughout the years, it has been utilized to prevent kidney transplant rejection, to prevent restenosis in drug eluting cardiac stents, and in treatments for cancer and tuberous sclerosis.

mTOR promotes cellular senescence by promoting protein synthesis and cell growth. It also negatively regulates the autophagy pathway. During the aging process, the increased activity of mTOR can increase abnormal proteins, which may lead to degeneration disease. A decrease in autophagy can cause an increase of damaged proteins and thus accelerate the progression of senescence. Inhibition of mTOR has consistently demonstrated extension of life span in many organisms including yeast, *Drosophila*, and mice [79, 80]. In 2006, Powers et al. reported that inhibition of the TOR pathway extended the life span of yeast [81]. mTOR inhibition can also increase resistance to environmental stress [82]. Treatment with rapamycin has been found to inhibit mTOR and decreases the activity of some senescent markers [77]. In 2013, an international workshop focused on interventions to slow the aging process discussed such drug interventions for chronic conditions and/or old age that can delay or prevent disease via inhibition of the mTOR pathway [83].

Future Directions

Researches continue to study the science of aging with the hopes of finding a solution to the pathologic processes of aging. Superoxide dismutase and catalase have been studied for years and have found to increase the life span in several species as well as increase resistance to oxidative stress [84]. T-bars or thibarbituric acid-reactant substances are used to test for end products of lipid peroxidation, or free radicals. These are increased in the aging process, and, therefore, assays of T-bars have been used as a marker for monitoring free radicals and aging [85]. Caloric restriction has been noted to improve lean body mass, decrease fat mass, and improve mood in human subjects. In animal models, it has been found to extend the life span and delay chronic diseases. Further research is being done to determine the exact amount of calories that can allow for the positive effects [86, 87]. Recently, a research team from the Scripps Research Institute identified a new class of drugs called senolytics that have demonstrated the following effects: slowing of the aging process, improving cardiac function, and extending life span in animal models. Further research is being done to explore such effects and to eventually determine clinical responses in humans.

References

1. Baillargeon J, Urban RJ, Ottenbacher KJ, Pierson KS, Goodwin JS. Trends in androgen prescribing in the United States, 2001 to 2011. JAMA Intern Med. 2013;173(15):1465–6.
2. Larsen PR, Kronenberg H, Melmed S, Polonsky K. Williams textbook of endocrinology. 10th ed. Philadelphia: W.B. Saunders Company.
3. Bhasin S, Jasuja R. Selective androgen receptor modulators (SARMs) as function promoting therapies. Curr Opin Clin Nutr Metab Care. 2009;12(3):232–40.
4. Finkelstein JS, Lee H, Burnett-Bowie SA, Pallais JC, Yu EW, Borges LF, Jones BF, Barry CV, Wulczyn KE, Thomas BJ, Leder BZ. Gonadal steroids and body composition, strength, and sexual function in men. N Engl J Med. 2013;369(11):1011–22.
5. Bremner WJ, Vitiello MV, Prinz PN. Loss of circadian rhythmicity in blood testosterone levels with aging in normal men. J Clin Endocrinol Metab. 1983;56(6):1278.
6. Davidson JM, Chen JJ, Crapo L, Gray GD, Greenleaf WJ, Catania JA. Hormonal changes and sexual function in aging men. J Clin Endocrinol Metab. 1983;57:71–7.
7. Orwoll E, Lambert LC, Marshall LM, Phipps K, Blank J, Barrett-Connor E, Cauley J, Ensrud K, Cummings S. Testosterone and estradiol among older men. J Clin Endocrinol Metab. 2006;91:1336–44.
8. Brawer MK. Testosterone replacement in men with andropause: an overview. Rev Urol. 2004;6(Suppl 6):S9–S15.
9. Travison TG, Araujo AB, O'Donnell AB, Kupelian V, McKinlay JB. A population-level decline in serum testosterone levels in American men. J Clin Endocrinol Metab. 2007;92(1):196–202.
10. Srinath R, Dobs A. Enobosarm (GTx-024, S-22): a potential treatment for cachexia. Future Oncol. 2014;10(2):187–94.
11. Marzette E, Leeuwenburgh C. Skeletal muscle apoptosis, sarcopenia and frailty at old age. Exp Gerontol. 2006;41(12):1234–8.
12. Narayanan R, Mohler ML, Bohl CE, Miller DD, Dalton JT. Selective androgen receptor modulators in preclinical and clinical development. Nucl Recept Signal. 2008;6:e010.
13. Gautier A, Bonnet F, Dubois S, Massart C, Grosheny C, Bachelot A, Aubè C, Balkau B, Ducluzeau PH. Associations between visceral adipose tissue, inflammation and sex steroid concentrations in men. Clin Enocrinol (Oxf). 2013;78(3):373–8.
14. Katznelson L, Finkelstein JS, Schoenfeld DA, Rosenthal DI, Anderson EJ, Klibanski A. Increase in bone density and lean body mass during testosterone administration in men with acquired hypogonadism. J Clin Endocrinol Metab. 1996;81(12):4358.
15. Kupelian V, Page ST, Araujo AB, Travison TG, Bremner WJ, McKinlay JB. Low sex hormone-binding globulin, total testosterone, and symptomatic androgen deficiency are associated with development of the metabolic syndrome in nonobese men. J Clin Endocrinol Metab. 2006;91(3):843.

16. Laaksonen DE, Niskanen L, Punnonen K, Nyysönen K, Tuomeainen TP, Volkonen VP, Salonen R, Salonen JT. Testosterone and sex hormone-binding globulin predict the metabolic syndrome and diabetes in middle-aged men. Diabetes Care. 2004;27(5):1036.
17. Nettleship JE, Jones RD, Channer KS, Jones TH. Testosterone and coronary artery disease. Front Horm Res. 2009;37:91–107.
18. Heller RF, Wheeler MJ, Micallef J, Miller NE, Lewis B. Relationship of high density lipoprotein cholesterol with total and free testosterone and sex hormone binding globulin. Acta Endocrinol. 1983;104(2):253–6.
19. Morris PD, Channer KS. Testosterone and cardiovascular disease in men. Asian J Androl. 2012;14(3):428–35.
20. Riggs BL, Wahner HW, Seeman E, Offord KP, Dunn WL, Mazess RB, Johnson KA, Melton LJ 3rd. Changes in bone mineral density of the proximal femur and spine with aging. Differences between the postmenopausal and senile osteoporosis syndromes. J Clin Invest. 1982; 70(4):716.
21. Moran JM, Martin RR, Pedrera-Canal M, Alonso-Terron J, Rodriguez-Velasco FJ, Pedrera-Zamorano JD. Low testosterone levels are associated with poor peripheral bone mineral density and quantitative bone ultrasound at phalanges and calcaneus in healthy elderly men. Biol Res Nurs. 2015;17(2):169–74.
22. LeBlanc ES, Nielson CM, Marshall LM, Lapidus JA, Barrett-Connor E, Ensrud KE, Hoffman AR, Laughlin G, Ohlsson C, Orwoll ES. Osteoporotic fractures in Men Study Group. The effects of serum testosterone, estradiol, and sex hormone binding globulin level on fracture risk in older men. J Clin Endocrinol Metab. 2009;94(9):3337–46.
23. Joshi D, van Schoor NM, de Rone W, Schaap LA, Comijs HC, Beekman AT, Lips P. Low free testosterone levels are associated with prevalence and incidence of depressive symptoms in older men. Clin Endocrinol. 2010;72(2):232.
24. Shores MM, Moceri VM, Sloan KL, Mastusmoto AM, Kivlahan DR. Low testosterone levels predict incident depressive illness in older men: effects of age and medical morbidity. J Clin Psychiatry. 2005;66(1):7–14.
25. Yeap BB. Hormonal changes and their impact on cognition and mental health of ageing men. Maturitas. 2014;79(2):227–35.
26. Moffat SD, Zonderman AB, Metter EJ, Blackman MR, Harman SM, Resnick SM. Longitudinal assessment of serum free testosterone concentration predicts memory performance and cognitive status in elderly men. J Clin Endocrinol Metab. 2002;87(11):5001–7.
27. Ottenbacher KJ, Oteenbacher ME, Ottenbacher AJ, Acha AA, Ostire GV. Androgen treatment and muscle strength in elderly men: a meta-analysis. J Am Geriatr Soc. 2006;54(11):1666–73.
28. Corona G, Maseroli E, Rastrelli G, Isidori AM, Sforza A, Mannucci E, Maggi M. Cardiovascular risk associated with testosterone-boosting medications: a systematic review and meta-analysis. Expert Opin Drug Saf. 2014;13(10):1327–51.
29. Snyder PJ, Peachey H, Hannoush P, Berlin JA, Loh L, Holmes JH, Dlewati A, Staley J, Santanna J, Kapoor SC, Attie MF, Haddad JG Jr, Strom BL. Effect of testosterone treatment on bone mineral density in men over 65 years of age. J Clin Endocrinol Metab. 1999;84(6):1966.
30. Kenny AM, Prestwood KM, Gruman CA, Marcello KM, Raisz LG. Effects of transdermal testosterone on bone and muscle in older men with low bioavailable testosterone levels. J Gerontol A Biol Sci. 2001;56(5):M266.
31. Amory JK, Watts NB, Easley KA, Sutton PR, Anawalt BD, Matsumoto AM, Bremner WJ, Tenover JL. Exogenous testosterone or testosterone with finasteride increases bone mineral density in older men with lower serum testosterone. J Clin Endocrinol Metab. 2004;89(2):503.
32. Tracz MJ, Sideras K, Boloña ER, Haddad RM, Kennedy CC, Uraga MV, Caples SM, Erwin PJ, Montori VM. Testosterone use in men and its effects on bone health. A systematic review and meta-analysis of randomized placebo-controlled trials. J Clin Endocrinol Metab. 2006;91(6):2011–6.
33. Shores MM, Kivlahan DR, Sadak TI, Li EJ, Matsumoto AM. A randomized, double-blind, placebo-controlled study of testosterone treatment in hypogonadal older men with subthreshold depression (dysthymia or minor depression). J Clin Pyschiatry. 2009;70(7):1009–16.

34. Wang C, Swedloff RS, Iranmanesh A, Dobs A, Snyder PJ, Cunningham G, Matsumoto AM, Weber T, Berman N. Transdermal testosterone gel improves sexual function, mood, muscle strength, and body composition parameters in hypogonadal men. Testosterone Gel Study Group. J Clin Endocrinol Metab. 2000;85:2839–53.
35. Seidman SN, Orr G, Raviv G, Levi R, Roose SP, Kravitz E, Amiaz R, Weiser M. Effects of testosterone replacement in middle-aged men with dysthymia: a randomized, placebo-controlled clinical trial. J Clin Psychopharmacol. 2009;29(3):216–21.
36. Janowsky JS, Oviatt SK, Orwoll ES. Testosterone influences spatial cognition in older men. Behav Neurosci. 1994;108(2):325–32.
37. Cherrier MM, Asthana S, Plymate S, Baker L, Matsumoto AM, Peskind E, Raskind MA, Brodkin K, Bremner W, Petrova A, LaTendresse S, Craft S. Testosterone supplementation improves spatial and verbal memory in healthy older men. Neurology. 2001;57:80–8.
38. Bhasin S, Cunningham GR, Hayes FJ, Matsumoto AM, Snyder PJ, Swerdloff RS, Motori VM. Testosterone therapy in adult men with androgen deficiency syndromes: an endocrine society clinical practice guideline. J Clin Endocrinol Metab. 2006;91(6):1995–2010.
39. Vigen R, O'Donnell CI, Barón AE, Grunwald GK, Maddox TM, Bradley SM, Barqawi A, Woning G, Wierman ME, Plomondon ME, Rumsfeld JS, Ho PM. Association of testosterone therapy with mortality, myocardial infarction, and stroke in men with low testosterone levels. JAMA. 2013;310(17):1829–36.
40. Borst SE, Shuster JJ, Zou B, Ye F, Jia H, Wokhlu A, Yarrow JF. Cardiovascular risks and elevation of serum DHT vary by route of testosterone administration: a systematic review and meta-analysis. BMC Med. 2014;23:211.
41. Calof OM, Singh AB, Lee ML, Kenny AM, Urban RJ, Tenover JL, Bhasin S. Adverse events associated with testosterone replacement in middle-aged and older men: a meta-analysis of randomized, placebo-controlled trials. J Gerontol A Biol Sci Med Sci. 2005;60:1451–7.
42. Borst SE, Yarrow JF. Injection of testosterone may be safe and more effective than transdermal administration for combating loss of muscle and bone in older men. Am J Physiol Endocrinol Metab. 2015;308(12):E1035–42.
43. Ramis MR, Esteban S, Miralles A, Tan DX, Reiter RJ. Caloric restriction, resveratrol and melatonin: role of SIRT1 and implications for aging and related-diseases. Mech Ageing Dev. 2015;146–148:28–41.
44. Frèmont L. Biological effects of resveratrol. Life Sci. 2000;66(8):663–73.
45. Liu B, Zhang X, Zhang W, Zhen H. New enlightenment of French paradox: resveratrol's potential for cancer chemoprevention and anti-cancer therapy. Cancer Biol Ther. 2007;6(12):1833–6.
46. Renaud S, de Lorgeril M. Wine, alcohol, platelets, and the French paradox for coronary heart disease. Lancet. 1992;339(8808):1523–6.
47. Singh CK, Liu X, Ahmad N. Resveratrol, in its natural combination in whole grape, for health promotion and disease management. Ann N Y Acad Sci. 2015;1348(1):150–60.
48. Dutt V, Gupta S, Dabur R, Injeti E, Mittal A. Skeletal muscle atrophy: potential therapeutic agents and their mechanisms of action. Pharmacol Res. 2015;99:86–100.
49. Wang DT, Yin Y, Yang YJ, Lv PJ, Shi Y, Lu L, Wei LB. Resveratrol prevents TNF-α-induced muscle atrophy via regulation of Akt/mTOR/FoxO1 signaling in C2C12 myotubes. Int Immunopharmacol. 2014;19:206–13.
50. Ayub A, Poulose N, Raju R. Resveratrol improves survival and prolongs life following hemorrhagic shock. Mol Med. 2015;21:305–12.
51. Zunino SJ, Peerson JM, Freytag TL, Breksa AP, Bonnel EL, Woodhouse LR, Storms DH. Dietary grape powder increases IL-1β and IL-6 production by lipopolysaccharide-activated monocytes and reduces plasma concentrations of large LDL and large LDL-cholesterol particles in obese humans. Br J Nutr. 2014;112(3):369–80.
52. Prior RL, Gu L, Wu X, Jacob RA, Sotoudeh G, Kader AA, Cook RA. Plasma antioxidant capacity changes following a meal as a measure of the ability of a food to alter in vivo antioxidant status. J Am Coll Nutr. 2007;26(2):170–81.

53. Nguyen AV, Martinez M, Stamos MJ, Moyer MP, Planutis K, Hope C, Holcombe RF. Results of a phase I pilot clinical trial examining the effect of plant-derived resveratrol and grape powder on Wnt pathway target gene expression in colonic mucosa and colon cancer. Cancer Manag Res. 2009;1:25–37.
54. Bhardwaj A, Sethi G, Vadhan-Raj S, Bueso-Ramos C, Takada Y, Garu U, Nair AS, Shishodia S, Aggarwal BB. Resveratrol inhibits proliferation, induces apoptosis, and overcomes chemoresistance through down-regulation of STAT3 and nuclear factor-kappaB-regulated anti-apoptotic and cell survival gene products in human multiple myeloma cells. Blood. 2007; 109(6):2293–302.
55. Popat R, Plesner T, Davies F, Cook G, Cook M, Elliott P, Jacobson E, Gumbleton T, Oakervee H, Cavenagh J. A phase 2 study of SRT501 (resveratrol) with bortezomib for patients with relapsed or refractory multiple myeloma. Br J Haematol. 2013;160(5):714–7.
56. Visioli F. The resveratrol fiasco. Pharmacol Res. 2014;90:87.
57. Cummings DE, Merriam GR. Growth hormone therapy in adults. Annu Rev Med. 2003;54:513–33.
58. Blackman MR, Sorkin JD, Münzer T, Bellantoni MF, Busby-Whitehead J, Stevens TE, Jayme J, O'Connor KG, Christmas C, Tobin JD, Stewart KJ, Cottrell E, St Clair C, Pabst KM, Harman SM. Growth hormone and sex steroid administration in healthy aged women and men: a randomized controlled trial. JAMA. 2002;288(18):2282–92.
59. Yuen KCJ, Chong LE, Rhoads SA. In: De Groot LJ, Beck-Peccoz P, Chrousos G, Dungan K, Grossman A, Hershman JM, Koch C, McLachlan R, New M, Rebar R, Singer F, Vinik A, Weickert MO, editors. Evaluation of adult growth hormone deficiency: current and future perspectives. SourceEndotext [Internet]. South Dartmouth (MA): MDText.com, Inc.; 2000–2013.
60. Corpas E, Harman SM, Blackman MR. Human growth hormone and human aging. Endocr Rev. 1993;14(1):20–39.
61. Kargi AY, Merriam GR. In: De Groot LJ, Beck-Peccoz P, Chrousos G, Dungan K, Grossman A, Hershman JM, Koch C, McLachlan R, New M, Rebar R, Singer F, Vinik A, Weickert MO, editors. Age-related changes in the growth hormone axis and growth hormone therapy in the elderly. SourceEndotext [Internet]. South Dartmouth: MDText.com, Inc.; 2000–2011.
62. O'Connor KG, Tobin JD, Harman SM, Plato CC, Roy TA, Sherman SS, Blackman MR. Serum levels of insulin-like growth factor-I are related to age and not to body composition in healthy women and men. J Gerontol A Biol Sci Med Sci. 1998;53(3):M176–82.
63. Pavlov EP, Harman SM, Merriam GR, Gelato MC, Blackman MR. Response of growth hormone (GH) and somatomedin-C to GH-releasing hormone in healthy aging me. J Clin Endocrinol Metab. 1986;62(3):595.
64. Iovino M, Monteleone P, Steardo L. Repetitive growth hormone-releasing hormone administration restores the attenuated growth hormone (GH) response to GH-releasing hormone testing in normal aging. J Clin Endocrinol Metab. 1989;69(4):910.
65. Rudman D, Feller AG, Nagraj HS, Gergans GA, Lalitha PY, Goldberg AF, Schlenker RA, Cohn L, Rudman IW, Mattson DE. Effects of human growth hormone in men over 60 years old. N Engl J Med. 1990;323(1):1–6.
66. Vitiello MV, Moe KE, Merriam GR, Mazzoni G, Buchner DH, Schwartz RS. Growth hormone releasing hormone improves the cognition of healthy older adults. Neurobiol Aging. 2006;27(2):318–23. Epub 2005 Mar 23
67. Rudman D, Feller AG, Cohn L, Shetty KR, Rudman IW, Draper MW. Effects of human growth hormone on body composition in elderly men. Horm Res. 1991;36(Suppl 1):73–81.
68. Appelman-Dijkstra NM, Claessen KM, Hamdy NA, Pereira AM, Biermasz NR. Effects of up to 15 years of recombinant human GH (rhGH) replacement on bone metabolism in adults with growth hormone deficiency (GHD): the Leiden Cohort Study. Clin Endocrinol. 2014;81(5):727–35.
69. Sonntag WE, Ramsey M, Carter CS. Growth hormone and insulin-like growth factor-1 (IGF-1) and their influence on cognitive aging. Ageing Res Rev. 2005;4(2):195–212.

70. Liu H, Bravata DM, Olkin I, Nayak S, Roberts B, Garber AM, Hoffman AR. Systematic review: the safety and efficacy of growth hormone in the healthy elderly. Ann Intern Med. 2007;146(2):104–15.
71. Stochholm K, Johannsson G. Reviewing the safety of GH replacement therapy in adults. Growth Hormon IGF Res. 2015;25(4):149–57.
72. Mohler ML, Bohl CE, Jones A, Coss CC, Narayanan R, He Y, Hwang DJ, Dalton JT, Miller DD. Nonsteroidal selective androgen receptor modulators (SARMs): dissociating the anabolic and androgenic activities of the androgen receptor for therapeutic benefit. J Med Chem. 2009;52(12):3597–617.
73. Bhasin S, Calof OM, Storer TW, Lee ML, Mazer NA, Jasuja R, Montori VM, Gao W, Dalton JT. Drug insight: testosterone and selective androgen receptor modulators as anabolic therapies for chronic illness and aging. Nat Clin Pract Endocrinol Metab. 2006;2(3):146–59.
74. Dobs AS, Boccia RV, Croot CC, Gabrail NY, Dalton JT, Hancock ML, Johnston MA, Steiner MS. Effects of enobosarm on muscle wasting and physical function in patients with cancer: a double-blind randomized controlled phase 2 trial. Lancet Oncol. 2013;14(4):335–45.
75. Dalton JT, Taylor RP, Mohler ML, Steiner MS. Selective androgen receptor modulators for the prevention and treatment of muscle wasting associated with cancer. Curr Opin Support Palliat Care. 2013;7(4):345–51.
76. Kearbey JD, Gao W, Narayanan R, Fisher SJ, Wu D, Miller DD, Dalton JT. Selective androgen receptor modulator (SARM) treatment prevents bone loss and reduces body fact in ovariectomized rats. Pharm Res. 2007;24(2):328–35.
77. Xu S, Cai Y, Wei Y. mTOR signaling from cellular senescence to organismal aging. Aging Dis. 2013;5(4):263–73.
78. Kaeberlein M. mTOR inhibition: from aging to autism and beyond. Scientifica (Cairo). 2013;2013:849186.
79. Miller RA, Harrison DE, Astle CM, Baur JA, Boyd AR, de Cabo R, Fernandez E, Flurkey K, Javors MA, Nelson JF, Orihuela CJ, Pletcher S, Sharp ZD, Sinclair D, Starnes JW, Wilkinson JE, Nadon NL, Strong R. Rapamycin, but not resveratrol or simvastatin, extends life span of genetically heterogeneous mice. J Gerontol A Biol Sci Med Sci. 2011;66(2):191–201.
80. Kaeberlein M. Rapamycin and ageing: when, for how long, and how much? J Genet Genomics. 2014;41(9):459–63.
81. Powers RW III, Kaeberlein M, Caldwell SD, Kennedy BK, Fields S. Extension of chronological life span in yeast by decreased TOR pathway signaling. Genes Dev. 2006;20(2):174–84.
82. Kenyon CJ. The genetics of ageing. Nature. 2010;464(7288):504–12.
83. Longo VD, Antebi A, Bartke A, Barzilai N, Brown-Borg HM, Caruso C, Curiel TJ, de Cabo R, Franceschi C, Gems D, Ingram DK, Johnson TE, Kennedy BK, Kenyon C, Klein S, Kopchick JJ, Lepperdinger G, Madeo F, Mirisola MG, Mitchell JR, Passarino G, Rudolph KL, Sedivy JM, Shadel GS, Sinclair DA, Spindler SR, Suh Y, Vijg J, Vinciguerra M, Fontana L. Interventions to slow aging in humans: are we ready? Aging Cell. 2015;14(4):497–510.
84. Warner HR. Superoxide dismutase, aging, and degenerative disease. Free Radic Biol Med. 1994;17(3):249–58.
85. Kawamoto EM, Vasconcelos AR, Degaspari S, Böhmer AE, Scavone C, Marcourakis T. Age-related changes in nitric oxide activity, cyclic GMP, and TBARS levels in platelets and erythrocytes reflect the oxidative status in central nervous system. Age (Dordr). 2013;35(2):331–42. https://doi.org/10.1007/s11357-011-9365-7. Epub 2012 Jan 26.
86. Heilbronn LK, Ravussin E. Calorie restriction and aging: review of the literature and implications for studies in humans. Am J Clin Nutr. 2003;78(3):361–9.
87. Kulkarni SS, Cantó C. The molecular targets of resveratrol. Biochim Biophys Acta. 2015; 1852(6):1114–23.

Chapter 7
Injectable, Biologics, and Stem Cells

Mitchell S. Fourman, Jay V. Kalawadia, and James Bradley

Pathophysiology of Osteoarthritis Pain

Joint pain related to osteoarthritis (OA) is often linked to an initial cartilage injury. Immunogenic cartilage breakdown products cause inflammation of the synovium, leading to the release of inflammatory markers and cytokines. Quiescent adult chondrocytes are subsequently activated, resulting in the further release of a host of inflammatory markers—most notably IL-1, IL-8, TNF-alpha, reactive oxygen species such as nitric oxide (NO), prostaglandins, matrix metalloproteinases, and leukotrienes [1–6]. This reaction leads to a breakdown of the cartilage matrix, chondrocyte apoptosis, and the activation of pain nociceptors within the cartilage, synovium, and subchondral bone [7]. This chronic inflammatory process can be viewed histologically, as synovial biopsies will demonstrate increased blood vessel proliferation, vascular endothelial growth factor (VEGF) expression, and increased mononuclear cell infiltration [8].

Pain within the osteoarthritic joint is unlikely to be immediately related to cartilage breakdown, as cartilage lacks nerve endings. However, the synovium, subchondral bone, and periosteum have dense concentrations of nociceptors [9]. Polymodal Aδ and C nociceptors include groups with low firing threshold for normal activity, while others maintain a high threshold for more injurious stimuli [10, 11]. A lesser-known third class is the sleeping nociceptor, which does not respond to typical pain stimuli, but instead to the endogenous stimuli from the injury itself. These in concert act to create the crescentic pain reaction typical in acute OA flares. An initial pain

M. S. Fourman, MD, MPhil · J. Bradley, MD (✉)
Department of Orthopaedic Surgery, University of Pittsburgh Medical Center,
Pittsburgh, PA, USA
e-mail: fourmanm@upmc.edu; bradleyjp@upmc.edu

J. V. Kalawadia, MD
Department of Orthopaedic Surgery, Orthopaedic Associates of Allentown, Allentown, PA, USA

© Springer International Publishing AG, part of Springer Nature 2018
V. J. Wright, K. K. Middleton (eds.), *Masterful Care of the Aging Athlete*,
https://doi.org/10.1007/978-3-319-16223-2_7

event may result in persistent hyperalgesia for years following the insult, leaving the patient prone to both central and peripheral sensitization [12, 13]. Resulting neuro-plasticity may be a strong contributor to the compounding pain complaint central to chronic osteoarthritis [14].

Different inflammatory cascades are required for each region of the joint to evoke a pain response. As such, the degree of pain related to synovial inflammation is location-specific. This is especially true in the knee, where inflammation around the infrapatellar fat pad has been correlated with increased pain [15]. Further evidence of synovial inflammation due to osteoarthritis includes synovial hyperplasia [16], lymphocytic infiltrate, fibrosis, and thickening of the synovial capsule [17, 18]. Synovial fibrosis in particular may be a primary contributor to joint pain and stiffness in OA [19]. Subchondral bone edema is one of the earliest observed signs of osteoarthritis, and bone marrow edema-like lesions (BML) can be seen on advanced imaging prior to the onset of clinical symptoms [20]. Areas of the sub-chondral bone with BMLs have been correlated with increased pain and cartilage erosion [21]. Current theory suggests that these BMLs allow for the rapid ingrowth of sensory fibers and vascular channels, leading to increased pain and sensitivity to inflammatory cytokines [22].

Nonsurgical Management of OA

While conservative management algorithms are often dictated by the individual physician, consensus guidelines for the management of osteoarthritis by the American College of Rheumatology (ACR) were released in 2012. These recommendations stratify patients by the severity and anatomic involvement of OA, specifically of the hand, hip, and knee.

Physical Therapy

The initial management of osteoarthritis includes targeted stretching and strengthening with physical therapy. Restrictive motion devices (i.e., splints, orthotics, braces, taping) for pain control and therapy guidance may provide relief to some patients although the literature demonstrates varying results on their efficacy [23, 24]. Similarly, aquatic exercise for the management of lower-extremity OA may help with pain relief and strengthening, although the global utility of these exercises has been inconsistently demonstrated among various studies [25–27]. For these reasons, the ACR does not recommend a specific exercise modality for hip or knee OA, but recommends tailored treatment based on the patient's aerobic capacity [23].

Several alternative therapies not included in consensus recommendations have been studied extensively. High-level evidence has demonstrated acupuncture to provide long-term pain relief for OA, comparable to exercise and off-loading modalities [28–30]. However, other studies demonstrated no significant improvement when compared to physical therapy [31]. Given this, the American Academy of Orthopaedic Surgery (AAOS) clinical guidelines state there is inconclusive proof of efficacy to fully support acupuncture [24]. Other alternative therapies such as yoga [32], massage [33, 34], and tai chi [35–37] have demonstrated varying levels of pain improvement for OA. The ACR does not provide any specific therapeutic recommendations, although acknowledges potential efficacy in patients with end-stage arthritis who are poor surgical candidates or deny surgical treatment [23].

Mild to Moderate OA: Pharmacologic Management

The initial therapy for OA includes non-narcotic analgesia and nonsteroidal anti-inflammatory (NSAID) drugs. Acetaminophen (paracetamol) has been found to decrease subjective pain scores by more than 4 on a 100-point scale when used as monotherapy and is, therefore, recommended as baseline analgesia for lower-extremity OA [38–40]. A maximum daily dose of 4000 mg/day may be taken. Topical capsaicin is recommended as concurrent first-line therapy in cases of hand OA [23]. However, the ACR notes that this recommendation is not based on any validated therapeutic benefit. A meta-analysis of mostly retrospective work found a modest but significant improvement in pain following 4 weeks of continuous use [41, 42]. Unfortunately, this was not observed in randomized controlled trials.

NSAID therapy is considered a second-line treatment for lower-extremity OA and may be administered concurrently with acetaminophen to provide supplemental pain relief [43]. Given the risk of upper gastrointestinal (GI) complications related to long-term NSAID use [44], the ACR recommends that patients with a history of GI complications or concurrently on a prescribed full-dose aspirin use a COX-2 selective inhibitor only or begin a proton pump inhibitor (i.e., pantoprazole) concurrently [23, 45, 46]. The therapeutic benefit of selective COX-2 inhibitors has been found to be equivalent to nonselective NSAIDs, with no difference in complication rate observed [47]. The ACR contraindicates NSAIDs for patients over the age of 75, in line with previously published recommendations by the American Geriatrics Society [48].

The ACR has few recommendations for non-injectable monotherapies in the case of OA pain refractory to acetaminophen and NSAIDs. Pain improvement with tramadol monotherapy has been inconsistently demonstrated. However, tramadol has shown benefit as an adjunct therapy [49]. Randomized controlled trials show significant improvement in the pain ratings of patients with moderate to severe OA when tramadol is administered in conjunction with acetaminophen or NSAIDs [50]. Findings suggest that the analgesic effects of tramadol with NSAIDs are synergistic.

Chondroitin Sulfate + Glucosamine

Chondroitin sulfate and glucosamine, an amino sugar and carbohydrate naturally found within healthy cartilage, have been commonly utilized as an alternative or supplemental therapy for osteoarthritis. Supporters believe the reduction in chondroitin sulfate concentration and chain length seen in OA can be exogenously replenished [51, 52]. Several clinical trials have focused on the clinical benefits of these supplements.

While available in injectable form, chondroitin sulfate and glucosamine are predominately taken orally [53]. Randomized controlled trials using chondroitin sulfate as an adjunct to NSAID therapy showed both pain and structural improvements, with a reduced loss of cartilage volume at a 2-year endpoint [54]. Additional studies have demonstrated a reduction in NSAID use and improvement in mobility with long-term glucosamine as well [55, 56]. While the conclusions of these clinical trials are encouraging, several other trials refuted their conclusions [57, 58]. A large randomized controlled trial evaluating chondroitin sulfate and glucosamine as both monotherapy and adjunct failed to show any improvement in a global cohort compared to NSAID therapy alone [59].

While randomized trials and high-quality meta-analyses have been attempted to study the benefit of chondroitin sulfate and glucosamine, the inconsistent dosage, preparation, and administration has made it difficult to demonstrate an irrefutable clinical benefit. For this reason, the ACR only recommends the use of these supplements as adjuncts to traditional pharmacologic therapies, while the AAOS does not recommend their usage at all [23, 24]. Given low toxicity of these drugs and over-the-counter availability, they remain popular alternative therapies for OA [60].

Opioids in Osteoarthritis

Consensus recommendations regarding the role opioids should play in the management of OA are inconclusive [24]. A Cochrane review noted a modest pain improvement with opioid therapy, but also noted a high rate of opioid abuse and addiction [61]. While objective pain improvements have failed to demonstrate clinical significance, the high patient perception of opioid efficacy in the USA complicates therapeutic guidance [62]. As such prescription rates of opioids are significantly higher in the USA than in Europe and elsewhere in the world [63, 64].

Injectable Treatments

Intra-articular Corticosteroids

Intra-articular corticosteroids injections (CSI) remain the mainstay of injectable clinical therapy for moderate to severe osteoarthritis. There exists conflicting evidence supporting their efficacy, and as such, official recommendations have often been inconclusive. Recent revisions of the ACR recommendations recommend CSI for those patients with soft tissue inflammation and joint effusion [23], although the AAOS clinical guidelines remain inconclusive [24]. Advantages of CSI include a rapid onset of action, significant long-term local anti-inflammatory effects, and a limited, although significant, risk of side effects [65, 66].

Mechanism of action: The onset of corticosteroid activity begins upon activation by the surface receptors of the synovial membrane. The activated corticosteroid acts on the nuclear steroid receptors directly, reducing the rate of mRNA and protein synthesis. This in turn inhibits the function of T and B cells as well as phospholipase A2 and, consequently, arachidonic acid [67, 68]. Besides inhibiting the pro-inflammatory milieu produced as a downstream effect of osteoarthritis progression, corticosteroids may further exert a disease-modifying role. In vivo animal studies suggest that CSI decrease the severity of osteophyte formation and cartilage fibrillations related to OA. These effects were observed in both prophylactic and therapeutic trials [69, 70].

Composition: Corticosteroid preparations are largely derivatives of prednisolone (Table 7.1). The creation of large particle suspensions poorly soluble in water, such as with triamcinolone acetonide, allows the drug to remain in the joint for a longer period and requires hydrolysis by cellular esterases to release its active component [72, 73]. However, the rate of cellular uptake is slow, leading to a delayed onset of effect [73]. In contrast, drugs that are "clear," or non-particulate, suspensions such as dexamethasone salt are rapidly taken up by cells and, therefore, are faster acting. However, the drug spends less time within the joint, theoretically reducing the duration of effect [73]. Recent clinical trials comparing ester and salt preparations have found that their efficacy and duration may be equivalent, suggesting that pharmacodynamics may not be of clinical significance [74]. Mixed preparations have not shown any benefit. A randomized trial assessing the benefit of a combination approach utilizing a mixture of the salt and ester forms of betamethasone has failed to show any improvement in duration or onset time with this approach compared to ester-only preparations [72, 75].

Efficacy: CSI have been shown to provide short- to mid-term pain relief in patients with OA [76]. Some evidence suggests that clinical improvement in pain and range of motion can be expected from 2 to 12 weeks post-injection, with an average reduction in pain score of over 20% [65, 77, 78]. A longer duration of efficacy has been demonstrated in patients with preexisting soft tissue involvement [79, 80], although soft tissue involvement in general had poorer therapeutic responses overall [81]. The long-term efficacy and safety of CSI remain a concern. Randomized trials in patients with knee OA suggest that regular injections every 3 months out to 2 years following initiation resulted in prolonged reductions in pain and stiffness [82].

Side effects: In addition to the side effect of transiently elevated blood glucose levels, particularly in diabetics, both local and systemic complications related to CSI have been described [83]. In vitro studies have demonstrated that direct exposure of corticosteroids to cartilage has a chondrotoxic effect [84, 85]. The clinical manifestation of this has yet to be determined. Skin atrophy, hypersensitivity, and hypopigmentation with a classic "linear ray" appearance have long been associated

Table 7.1 Solubility and molecular characteristics of common corticosteroid preparations [71]

Steroid	Commercial names	Equivalent potency (mg)	Solubility	Maximum particle size (μm)	Particles >10 μm (%)	Particle aggregation	Benzyl alcohol	Polyethylene glycol
Methylprednisolone acetate	Depo-Medrol, Solu-Medrol, Duralone, Medralone	4	0.001	>500	45	Few	Yes	Yes
Triamcinolone acetonide	Kenalog	4	0.0002	>500	45	Extensive	Yes	No
Betamethasone acetate, betamethasone sodium phosphate	Celestone Soluspan, Betaject	0.75	Acetate form: "practically insoluble"; sodium phosphate form: Freely soluble	500	35	Some	No	No
Dexamethasone sodium phosphate	Decadron Phosphate, Adrenocot, Decaject	0.75	Freely soluble	0.5	0	None	Yes	No

Referenced from: MacMahon, P.J., S.J. Eustace, and E.C. Kavanagh, Injectable corticosteroid and local anesthetic preparations: a review for radiologists. Radiology. 2009. 252(3): p. 647–61 with intralesional or intra-articular steroid therapy. The mechanism behind this clinical manifestation is not fully understood, although current theory suggests that the lymphatic system may play an important role [86]. Tendon rupture and in vitro cellular degeneration following exposure to corticosteroids have been reported. While this mechanism is also poorly understood, recent findings suggest that increased apoptosis, transient increases in matrix metalloproteinases (e.g., MMP-3), and an active inhibition of repair mechanisms may be important contributors to tendon degeneration [87–89].

Viscosupplementation

In the pro-inflammatory arthritic cascade, the synovial fluid undergoes several compositional changes. Synovial fluid, traditionally responsible for the lubrication and smooth motion of joints, functions due to the presence of hyaluronate. Hyaluronate, a high-molecular-mass polysaccharide, gives synovial fluid its abilities to act as shock absorber and lubricant medium. In the osteoarthritic joint, the amount and quality of hyaluronate are both decreased, in part due to increased degradation rates. There is some evidence that the degradation of synovial fluid may be slowed or reversed with viscosupplementation.

Mechanism of action: Viscosupplementation exerts a anti-inflammatory effect on synovium, inhibiting the release of prostaglandins and the immunologic response typical in osteoarthritis [90]. Further theories suggesting that cartilage degeneration may be reversed with viscosupplementation have not borne out conclusively in the literature.

Composition: Current formulations of hyaluronic acid vary in molecular weight to modulate elastoviscosity. High-molecular-weight formulations, such as the well-tested hylan G-F-20, will have higher elastoviscosity compared to low-molecular-weight preparations. This property appears to be critical to the therapeutic effect of viscosupplementation, with an initial randomized trial showing that hylan G-F-20 improved pain and patient reported outcomes compared to low-molecular-weight preparations [91]. However, subsequent trials have been inconsistent in replicating this finding [92]. Moreover, studies in animal models suggest that high-molecular-weight hyaluronic acid may be more effective at binding to its cellular receptor and as a result more effective at reducing synovial inflammation and stabilizing synovial fluid [93].

Efficacy: Randomized controlled trials and meta-analysis exhibit significant variability and disagreement as to the efficacy of viscosupplementation. In general, many randomized controlled trials suggest that viscosupplementation is associated with some degree of pain relief in osteoarthritis patients. However, the degree and duration of pain relief is a source of disagreement. In general, trials agree that the longest expected efficacy of viscosupplementation is 5–6 months [94, 95], although Campbell et al. [96] found no improvement at any time point. Benefits beyond pain have also been proposed, with improvements demonstrated in gait kinematics following a course of viscosupplementation [97].

Viscosupplementation has traditionally been given in three separate weekly injections. However, this methodology has not been well validated in the literature, with randomized trials finding no significant clinical differences between three separate injections compared to one alone [98]. Given the disparate evidence, while some consensus opinions suggest that viscosupplementation may be of some clinical benefit, they do not establish guidelines for its use as differing trial metrics make comparison difficult [99]. The AAOS does not recommend viscosupplementation given the lack of conclusive evidence [24].

Side effects: Proponents of viscosupplementation have pointed to its low toxicity and paucity of side effects. Meta-analyses have demonstrated that viscosupplementation is safe, with an increased risk of minor adverse effect rate of less than 1% [100]. Reported complications include pseudosepsis secondary to an exaggerated immune reaction against a component of hyaluronic acid with higher rates found in avian-derived viscosupplementation products [101].

Platelet-Rich Plasma (PRP)

Mechanism of action: The beneficial mechanism behind a platelet concentrate compared with the injection of pure activated growth factor is not fully understood. However, recent in vitro studies suggest that there is a new class of cytokines present only in platelets, dedicated toward inflammatory regulation, protecting host tissues, and promoting angiogenesis [102]. Early studies on the impact of exogenous PRP on chemotaxis showed an increase in pro-inflammatory IL-1β, as well as phenotypic conversion of neutrophils and monocytes. Following this pro-inflammatory state, PRP may influence the expression of growth factors such as VEGF, TGF-β, and hepatocyte growth factor (HGF), which in turn inhibit the NF-κB inflammatory cascade. This may ultimately lead to an induction of immunologic quiescence, improving the inflammatory cascade seen in osteoarthritic joints. This immunologic quiescence has also been associated with the in vitro restoration of collagen-2 and aggrecan function around collagen scaffolds. Further functions of PRP include angiogenic proliferation via alpha-granules, although the balance between PRP-induced blood vessel growth and regression is not fully understood. PRP is also noted for other potentially chondroprotective functions, mediated via matrix metalloproteinases, alpha-2-macroglobulins, and overexpression of TGF-β.

Composition: Inconsistency in the preparation and delivery of PRP has made it difficult to study its efficacy. Currently, there are no standardized recommendations for the preparation of PRP. It is therefore often influenced by the experience and decision-making of the practitioner, the cost of the system in both time and laboratory expense, and the nature of the individual patient.

PRP is created when whole blood extracted from the patient is spun down in a centrifuge, removing red blood cells. There are multiple techniques currently employed to perform blood centrifugation, and a description of each is beyond the scope of this chapter. However, depending on the method of preparation, the platelet concentration and leukocyte levels will vary. Whether leukocytes should be removed from the platelet concentrate is not fully understood. Leukocyte-poor preparations may be beneficial in pro-inflammatory processes such as osteoarthritis; leukocyte-rich preparations may be better suited for chronic tendinopathy. Simplifying biology, platelets are anabolic sources, while leukocytes are catabolic. While one would expect leukocytes to counteract the benefit of a platelet concentrate, this has not been fully demonstrated [103]. Concentrates that contain leukocytes are labeled "L-PRP," while pure platelet concentrate is "P-PRP." The timing of PRP "activation" is not fully standardized and is also a product of individual technique. Pre-activation of platelets is stimulated with calcium chloride or thrombin introduced prior to injection. In contrast, postinjection activation is accomplished by endogenous tissue factors.

Efficacy: Studies evaluating the objective efficacy of PRP on osteoarthritic pain and function are varied. Multiple studies comparing a series of three weekly injections of exogenously activated P-PRP with viscosupplementation showed a significant improvement in pain, stiffness, and functional capacity at 5 weeks following the initiation of therapy [104, 105]. Gobbi et al. [106] noted improvement in symptoms beyond 1 year after administration. Other studies, however, have failed to corroborate these findings. Filardo et al. [107] found an improvement among younger patients with mild osteoarthritis, but their subsequent study failed to find any evidence of the superiority of PRP over viscosupplementation [108]. In those studies that reported clinical improvement, consistencies included PRP that underwent at least two centrifugations, at least two injections spaced by 1 week, and exogenous activation [109].

Collectively, the science surrounding PRP is in the infantile stages. Of the studies that exist, the methodologies are significantly varied, making generalizations difficult and meta-analyses limited [110]. Within the last few years, increasing evidence supports the formulation of PRP plays a substantial role as to its efficacy. Several factors exist within the PRP such as platelet-derived growth factor (PDGF), transforming growth factor (TGF), vascular endothelial growth factor (VEGF), fibroblast growth factor (FGF), interleukin-1 (IL-1), and matrix metalloproteinase-9 (MMP-9) depending on the preparation used [111]. These molecules in the proper concentrations have been shown to protect and heal cartilage [112]. Leukocyte-rich versus leukocyte-poor PRP has been suspected to matter as well. As research is suggesting the exact composition of PRP matters, it calls into question the results of early studies which did not take PRP creation, composition, or concentration into account. Further research is needed to identify the effects of the components of PRP and produce standardized formulations in order to study its clinical efficacy [113, 114]. As such, the current AAOS consensus recommendation on PRP remain inconclusive [24].

Side effects: Side effects related to PRP therapy may be related to both preparation and host factors. In a comparison of single and double spinning of PRP, a greater incidence of swelling and local pain reaction were noted in the double spun sample [104]. This was consistent between both L-PRP and P-PRP [103]. All side effects were transient and did not change long-term clinical outcomes. Additional basic science and clinical studies are needed to further define the mechanisms of action and side effect profiles of PRP therapies. Various compositions of PRP and a lack of well-known mechanisms of action pose important challenges to evaluating its efficacy, determining its adverse effects profile, and thus standardizing its use.

Stem Cell Therapy

While many cell types have been tested as a potential therapy for osteoarthritis and other musculoskeletal pathologies, bone marrow-derived stromal cells (BMSCs) appear prominently in the literature and are best understood.

Mechanism of action: The mechanism of action of BMSCs is thought to be through the induction of a chondroprotective cascade consisting of anti-inflammatory, antiapoptotic, and immunosuppressive functions, thereby permitting cartilage regeneration. Systemic mediators are key to chondrocyte differentiation and include parathyroid hormone-like peptide and basic fibroblast growth factor (FGF).

Composition: Given the lack of regulatory guidance on stem call preparation, delivery technique is variable. In the case of BMSCs, cells are typically isolated via bone marrow aspiration from the iliac crest. Cells are spun down to a concentrate in a manner similar to PRP, followed by resuspension in culture medium. These cells may be utilized immediately, or frozen in liquid nitrogen for later use. The stem cell quantity or concentration needed for therapeutic effect is variable, as is the way in which they are delivered into the osteoarthritic joint. Previously published mechanisms for stem cell delivery range from BMSCs loaded onto a scaffold [115] to the direct injection of incubated BMSCs [116]. As the cellular environment has been shown to be critical, most preparations are suspended within a growth factor-rich milieu. Human studies have utilized 1–12 million cell count preparations, and the exact cell concentration and count is inconsistently reported and varies widely. How the cells are cultured and how they are delivered remain an evolving research topic.

Efficacy: Studies utilizing autologous BMSC injection are generally encouraging, although irregularities related to stem cell composition and preparation complicate the interpretation of findings. A close examination of the cartilage defects post-injection in an in vivo rat model shows evidence of hypertrophic hyaline-like cartilage growth [117]. A synergy of BMSC therapy with PRP and physical therapy has been suggested, with synergistic improvement in patient reported knee and quality-of-life scores [118]. Allogeneic delivery of cultured BMSCs has also shown promising early findings. A randomized controlled trial delivering 40 million allogeneic BMSCs showed a significant increase in pain and function over the 1-year trial period [119]. While these early studies are encouraging, the lack of high-quality trials and the lack of standardized preparation protocols complicate a full assessment of the benefits of BMSC therapy [120]. As a result, the AAOS currently has no consensus opinion on stem cell therapy for osteoarthritis [24].

Side effects: There is a paucity of reported complications when utilizing stem cell therapy other than donor site morbidity. Long-term outcomes within knees and shoulders and with a matrix preparation have not been studied extensively owing to the recent development of stem cell technology. Well-powered randomized controlled trials examining stem cell therapy will be needed as the field develops.

References

1. Hardy MM, Seibert K, Manning PT, et al. Cyclooxygenase 2-dependent prostaglandin E2 modulates cartilage proteoglycan degradation in human osteoarthritis explants. Arthritis Rheum. 2002;46(7):1789–803.
2. Lee AS, Ellman MB, Yan D, et al. A current review of molecular mechanisms regarding osteoarthritis and pain. Gene. 2013;527(2):440–7.
3. Bian Q, Wang YJ, Liu SF, et al. Osteoarthritis: genetic factors, animal models, mechanisms, and therapies. Front Biosci (Elite Ed). 2012;4:74–100.
4. Fernandes JC, Martel-Pelletier J, Pelletier JP. The role of cytokines in osteoarthritis pathophysiology. Biorheology. 2002;39(1–2):237–46.
5. Goldring MB, Berenbaum F. The regulation of chondrocyte function by proinflammatory mediators: prostaglandins and nitric oxide. Clin Orthop Relat Res. 2004;(427 Suppl):S37–46.
6. Eyre DR, McDevitt CA, Billingham ME, et al. Biosynthesis of collagen and other matrix proteins by articular cartilage in experimental osteoarthrosis. Biochem J. 1980;188(3):823–37.
7. Im HJ, Li X, Muddasani P, et al. Basic fibroblast growth factor accelerates matrix degradation via a neuro-endocrine pathway in human adult articular chondrocytes. J Cell Physiol. 2008;215(2):452–63.
8. Goldring MB. Osteoarthritis and cartilage: the role of cytokines. Curr Rheumatol Rep. 2000;2(6):459–65.
9. Hunter DJ, McDougall JJ, Keefe FJ. The symptoms of OA and the genesis of pain. Rheum Dis Clin N Am. 2008;34(3):623–43.
10. Grigg P, Schaible HG, Schmidt RF. Mechanical sensitivity of group III and IV afferents from posterior articular nerve in normal and inflamed cat knee. J Neurophysiol. 1986;55(4):635–43.
11. Schaible HG, Schmidt RF. Effects of an experimental arthritis on the sensory properties of fine articular afferent units. J Neurophysiol. 1985;54(5):1109–22.
12. Coderre TJ, Katz J, Vaccarino AL, et al. Contribution of central neuroplasticity to pathological pain: review of clinical and experimental evidence. Pain. 1993;52(3):259–85.
13. Gwilym SE, Keltner JR, Warnaby CE, et al. Psychophysical and functional imaging evidence supporting the presence of central sensitization in a cohort of osteoarthritis patients. Arthritis Rheum. 2009;61(9):1226–34.
14. Melzack R, Coderre TJ, Katz J, et al. Central neuroplasticity and pathological pain. Ann N Y Acad Sci. 2001;933:157–74.
15. Ballegaard C, Riis RG, Bliddal H, et al. Knee pain and inflammation in the infrapatellar fat pad estimated by conventional and dynamic contrast-enhanced magnetic resonance imaging in obese patients with osteoarthritis: a cross-sectional study. Osteoarthr Cartil. 2014;22(7):933–40.
16. Hill CL, Gale DG, Chaisson CE, et al. Knee effusions, popliteal cysts, and synovial thickening: association with knee pain in osteoarthritis. J Rheumatol. 2001;28(6):1330–7.
17. Roach HI, Aigner T, Soder S, et al. Pathobiology of osteoarthritis: pathomechanisms and potential therapeutic targets. Curr Drug Targets. 2007;8(2):271–82.
18. Aigner T, Sachse A, Gebhard PM, et al. Osteoarthritis: pathobiology-targets and ways for therapeutic intervention. Adv Drug Deliv Rev. 2006;58(2):128–49.
19. Remst DF, Blaney Davidson EN, van der Kraan PM. Unravelling osteoarthritis-related synovial fibrosis: a step closer to solving joint stiffness. Rheumatology (Oxford). 2015;54:1954.
20. Felson DT, Niu J, Guermazi A, et al. Correlation of the development of knee pain with enlarging bone marrow lesions on magnetic resonance imaging. Arthritis Rheum. 2007;56(9):2986–92.
21. Felson DT, Chaisson CE, Hill CL, et al. The association of bone marrow lesions with pain in knee osteoarthritis. Ann Intern Med. 2001;134(7):541–9.
22. Wood JN. Nerve growth factor and pain. N Engl J Med. 2010;363(16):1572–3.
23. Hochberg MC, Altman RD, April KT, et al. American College of Rheumatology 2012 recommendations for the use of nonpharmacologic and pharmacologic therapies in osteoarthritis of the hand, hip, and knee. Arthritis Care Res (Hoboken). 2012;64(4):465–74.
24. Jevsevar DS, Brown GA, Jones DL, et al. The American Academy of Orthopaedic Surgeons evidence-based guideline on: treatment of osteoarthritis of the knee, 2nd edition. J Bone Joint Surg Am. 2013;95(20):1885–6.

25. Lu M, Su Y, Zhang Y, et al. Effectiveness of aquatic exercise for treatment of knee osteoarthritis: systematic review and meta-analysis. Z Rheumatol. 2015;74(6):543–52.
26. Bressel E, Wing JE, Miller AI, et al. High-intensity interval training on an aquatic treadmill in adults with osteoarthritis: effect on pain, balance, function, and mobility. J Strength Cond Res. 2014;28(8):2088–96.
27. Waller B, Ogonowska-Slodownik A, Vitor M, et al. Effect of therapeutic aquatic exercise on symptoms and function associated with lower limb osteoarthritis: systematic review with meta-analysis. Phys Ther. 2014;94(10):1383–95.
28. Ashraf A, Zarei F, Hadianfard MJ, et al. Comparison the effect of lateral wedge insole and acupuncture in medial compartment knee osteoarthritis: a randomized controlled trial. Knee. 2014;21(2):439–44.
29. Manheimer E, Linde K, Lao L, et al. Meta-analysis: acupuncture for osteoarthritis of the knee. Ann Intern Med. 2007;146(12):868–77.
30. Kwon YD, Pittler MH, Ernst E. Acupuncture for peripheral joint osteoarthritis: a systematic review and meta-analysis. Rheumatology (Oxford). 2006;45(11):1331–7.
31. Foster NE, Thomas E, Barlas P, et al. Acupuncture as an adjunct to exercise based physiotherapy for osteoarthritis of the knee: randomised controlled trial. BMJ. 2007;335(7617):436.
32. Garfinkel MS, Schumacher HR Jr, Husain A, et al. Evaluation of a yoga based regimen for treatment of osteoarthritis of the hands. J Rheumatol. 1994;21(12):2341–3.
33. Perlman AI, Sabina A, Williams AL, et al. Massage therapy for osteoarthritis of the knee: a randomized controlled trial. Arch Intern Med. 2006;166(22):2533–8.
34. Yip YB, Tam AC. An experimental study on the effectiveness of massage with aromatic ginger and orange essential oil for moderate-to-severe knee pain among the elderly in Hong Kong. Complement Ther Med. 2008;16(3):131–8.
35. Kang JW, Lee MS, Posadzki P, et al. T'ai chi for the treatment of osteoarthritis: a systematic review and meta-analysis. BMJ Open. 2011;1(1):e000035.
36. Wang C, Schmid CH, Hibberd PL, et al. Tai chi is effective in treating knee osteoarthritis: a randomized controlled trial. Arthritis Rheum. 2009;61(11):1545–53.
37. Ni GX, Song L, Yu B, et al. Tai chi improves physical function in older Chinese women with knee osteoarthritis. J Clin Rheumatol. 2010;16(2):64–7.
38. Chou R. Review: acetaminophen reduces pain in hip or knee osteoarthritis by a small amount, but not low back pain. Ann Intern Med. 2015;163(2):Jc10.
39. Verkleij SP, Luijsterburg PA, Bohnen AM, et al. NSAIDs vs acetaminophen in knee and hip osteoarthritis: a systematic review regarding heterogeneity influencing the outcomes. Osteoarthr Cartil. 2011;19(8):921–9.
40. Towheed TE, Maxwell L, Judd MG, et al. Acetaminophen for osteoarthritis. Cochrane Database Syst Rev. 2006;(1):CD004257.
41. Laslett LL, Jones G. Capsaicin for osteoarthritis pain. Prog Drug Res. 2014;68:277–91.
42. McCarthy GM, McCarty DJ. Effect of topical capsaicin in the therapy of painful osteoarthritis of the hands. J Rheumatol. 1992;19(4):604–7.
43. Makris UE, Abrams RC, Gurland B, et al. Management of persistent pain in the older patient: a clinical review. JAMA. 2014;312(8):825–36.
44. Lanas A, Boers M, Nuevo J. Gastrointestinal events in at-risk patients starting non-steroidal anti-inflammatory drugs (NSAIDs) for rheumatic diseases: the EVIDENCE study of European routine practice. Ann Rheum Dis. 2015;74(4):675–81.
45. Richette P, Latourte A, Frazier A. Safety and efficacy of paracetamol and NSAIDs in osteoarthritis: which drug to recommend? Expert Opin Drug Saf. 2015;14(8):1259–68.
46. Sostek MB, Fort JG, Estborn L, et al. Long-term safety of naproxen and esomeprazole magnesium fixed-dose combination: phase III study in patients at risk for NSAID-associated gastric ulcers. Curr Med Res Opin. 2011;27(4):847–54.
47. Angiolillo DJ, Datto C, Raines S, et al. Impact of concomitant low-dose aspirin on the safety and tolerability of naproxen and esomeprazole magnesium delayed-release tablets in patients requiring chronic nonsteroidal anti-inflammatory drug therapy: an analysis from 5 phase III studies. J Thromb Thrombolysis. 2014;38(1):11–23.

48. American Geriatrics Society Panel on Pharmacological Management of Persistent Pain in Older Persons. Pharmacological management of persistent pain in older persons. J Am Geriatr Soc. 2009;57(8):1331–46.
49. Dhillon S. Tramadol/paracetamol fixed-dose combination: a review of its use in the management of moderate to severe pain. Clin Drug Investig. 2010;30(10):711–38.
50. Silverfield JC, Kamin M, Wu SC, et al. Tramadol/acetaminophen combination tablets for the treatment of osteoarthritis flare pain: a multicenter, outpatient, randomized, double-blind, placebo-controlled, parallel-group, add-on study. Clin Ther. 2002;24(2):282–97.
51. Ishimaru D, Sugiura N, Akiyama H, et al. Alterations in the chondroitin sulfate chain in human osteoarthritic cartilage of the knee. Osteoarthr Cartil. 2014;22(2):250–8.
52. Bruyere O, Reginster JY. Glucosamine and chondroitin sulfate as therapeutic agents for knee and hip osteoarthritis. Drugs Aging. 2007;24(7):573–80.
53. Rivera F, Bertignone L, Grandi G, et al. Effectiveness of intra-articular injections of sodium hyaluronate-chondroitin sulfate in knee osteoarthritis: a multicenter prospective study. J Orthop Traumatol. 2016;17(1):27–33.
54. Martel-Pelletier J, Roubille C, Abram F, et al. First-line analysis of the effects of treatment on progression of structural changes in knee osteoarthritis over 24 months: data from the osteoarthritis initiative progression cohort. Ann Rheum Dis. 2015;74(3):547–56.
55. Rovati LC, Girolami F, D'Amato M, et al. Effects of glucosamine sulfate on the use of rescue non-steroidal anti-inflammatory drugs in knee osteoarthritis: results from the Pharmaco-Epidemiology of GonArthroSis (PEGASus) study. Semin Arthritis Rheum. 2016;45(4 Suppl):S34–41.
56. Kanzaki N, Ono Y, Shibata H, et al. Glucosamine-containing supplement improves locomotor functions in subjects with knee pain: a randomized, double-blind, placebo-controlled study. Clin Interv Aging. 2015;10:1743–53.
57. Sawitzke AD, Shi H, Finco MF, et al. The effect of glucosamine and/or chondroitin sulfate on the progression of knee osteoarthritis: a report from the glucosamine/chondroitin arthritis intervention trial. Arthritis Rheum. 2008;58(10):3183–91.
58. Fransen M, Agaliotis M, Nairn L, et al. Glucosamine and chondroitin for knee osteoarthritis: a double-blind randomised placebo-controlled clinical trial evaluating single and combination regimens. Ann Rheum Dis. 2015;74(5):851–8.
59. Clegg DO, Reda DJ, Harris CL, et al. Glucosamine, chondroitin sulfate, and the two in combination for painful knee osteoarthritis. N Engl J Med. 2006;354(8):795–808.
60. Sawitzke AD, Shi H, Finco MF, et al. Clinical efficacy and safety of glucosamine, chondroitin sulphate, their combination, celecoxib or placebo taken to treat osteoarthritis of the knee: 2-year results from GAIT. Ann Rheum Dis. 2010;69(8):1459–64.
61. Hitzeman N, Athale N. Opioids for osteoarthritis of the knee or hip. Am Fam Physician. 2010;81(9):1094.
62. Posnett J, Dixit S, Oppenheimer B, et al. Patient preference and willingness to pay for knee osteoarthritis treatments. Patient Prefer Adherence. 2015;9:733–44.
63. Wilson N, Sanchez-Riera L, Morros R, et al. Drug utilization in patients with OA: a population-based study. Rheumatology (Oxford). 2015;54(5):860–7.
64. Solomon DH, Avorn J, Wang PS, et al. Prescription opioid use among older adults with arthritis or low back pain. Arthritis Care Res. 2006;55(1):35–41.
65. Bellamy N, Campbell J, Robinson V, et al. Intraarticular corticosteroid for treatment of osteoarthritis of the knee. Cochrane Database Syst Rev. 2006;(2):CD005328.
66. Hepper CT, Halvorson JJ, Duncan ST, et al. The efficacy and duration of intra-articular corticosteroid injection for knee osteoarthritis: a systematic review of level I studies. J Am Acad Orthop Surg. 2009;17(10):638–46.
67. Creamer P. Intra-articular corticosteroid injections in osteoarthritis: do they work and if so, how? Ann Rheum Dis. 1997;56(11):634–6.
68. D'Acquisto F, Paschalidis N, Raza K, et al. Glucocorticoid treatment inhibits annexin-1 expression in rheumatoid arthritis CD4+ T cells. Rheumatology (Oxford). 2008;47(5): 636–9.

69. Pelletier JP, DiBattista JA, Raynauld JP, et al. The in vivo effects of intraarticular corticosteroid injections on cartilage lesions, stromelysin, interleukin-1, and oncogene protein synthesis in experimental osteoarthritis. Lab Investig. 1995;72(5):578–86.
70. Pelletier JP, Martel-Pelletier J. In vivo protective effects of prophylactic treatment with tiaprofenic acid or intraarticular corticosteroids on osteoarthritic lesions in the experimental dog model. J Rheumatol Suppl. 1991;27:127–30.
71. MacMahon PJ, Eustace SJ, Kavanagh EC. Injectable corticosteroid and local anesthetic preparations: a review for radiologists. Radiology. 2009;252(3):647–61.
72. Blankenbaker DG, De Smet AA, Stanczak JD, et al. Lumbar radiculopathy: treatment with selective lumbar nerve blocks--comparison of effectiveness of triamcinolone and betamethasone injectable suspensions. Radiology. 2005;237(2):738–41.
73. Wright JM, Cowper JJ, Page Thomas DP, et al. The hydrolysis of cortisol 21-esters by a homogenate of inflamed rabbit synovium and by rheumatoid synovial fluid. Clin Exp Rheumatol. 1983;1(2):137–41.
74. Lomonte AB, de Morais MG, de Carvalho LO, et al. Efficacy of triamcinolone hexacetonide versus methylprednisolone acetate intraarticular injections in knee osteoarthritis: a randomized, double-blinded, 24-week study. J Rheumatol. 2015;42:1677.
75. Stanczak J, Blankenbaker DG, De Smet AA, et al. Efficacy of epidural injections of Kenalog and Celestone in the treatment of lower back pain. AJR Am J Roentgenol. 2003;181(5):1255–8.
76. Hirsch G, Kitas G, Klocke R. Intra-articular corticosteroid injection in osteoarthritis of the knee and hip: factors predicting pain relief—a systematic review. Semin Arthritis Rheum. 2013;42(5):451–73.
77. Godwin M, Dawes M. Intra-articular steroid injections for painful knees. Systematic review with meta-analysis. Can Fam Physician. 2004;50:241–8.
78. Yavuz U, Sokucu S, Albayrak A, et al. Efficacy comparisons of the intraarticular steroidal agents in the patients with knee osteoarthritis. Rheumatol Int. 2012;32(11):3391–6.
79. Kruse DW. Intraarticular cortisone injection for osteoarthritis of the hip. Is it effective? Is it safe? Curr Rev Musculoskelet Med. 2008;1(3–4):227–33.
80. Kullenberg B, Runesson R, Tuvhag R, et al. Intraarticular corticosteroid injection: pain relief in osteoarthritis of the hip? J Rheumatol. 2004;31(11):2265–8.
81. Chao J, Wu C, Sun B, et al. Inflammatory characteristics on ultrasound predict poorer long-term response to intraarticular corticosteroid injections in knee osteoarthritis. J Rheumatol. 2010;37(3):650–5.
82. Raynauld JP, Buckland-Wright C, Ward R, et al. Safety and efficacy of long-term intraarticular steroid injections in osteoarthritis of the knee: a randomized, double-blind, placebo-controlled trial. Arthritis Rheum. 2003;48(2):370–7.
83. Habib G, Safia A. The effect of intra-articular injection of betamethasone acetate/betamethasone sodium phosphate on blood glucose levels in controlled diabetic patients with symptomatic osteoarthritis of the knee. Clin Rheumatol. 2009;28(1):85–7.
84. Syed HM, Green L, Bianski B, et al. Bupivacaine and triamcinolone may be toxic to human chondrocytes: a pilot study. Clin Orthop Relat Res. 2011;469(10):2941–7.
85. Dragoo JL, Danial CM, Braun HJ, et al. The chondrotoxicity of single-dose corticosteroids. Knee Surg Sports Traumatol Arthrosc. 2012;20(9):1809–14.
86. Venkatesan P, Fangman WL. Linear hypopigmentation and cutaneous atrophy following intra-articular steroid injections for de Quervain's tendonitis. J Drugs Dermatol. 2009;8(5):492–3.
87. Tempfer H, Gehwolf R, Lehner C, et al. Effects of crystalline glucocorticoid triamcinolone acetonide on cultered human supraspinatus tendon cells. Acta Orthop. 2009;80(3):357–62.
88. Muto T, Kokubu T, Mifune Y, et al. Temporary inductions of matrix metalloprotease-3 (MMP-3) expression and cell apoptosis are associated with tendon degeneration or rupture after corticosteroid injection. J Orthop Res. 2014;32(10):1297–304.
89. Hossain MA, Park J, Choi SH, et al. Dexamethasone induces apoptosis in proliferative canine tendon cells and chondrocytes. Vet Comp Orthop Traumatol. 2008;21(4):337–42.

90. Hunter DJ. Viscosupplementation for osteoarthritis of the knee. N Engl J Med. 2015;372(26):2570.
91. Wobig M, Bach G, Beks P, et al. The role of elastoviscosity in the efficacy of viscosupplementation for osteoarthritis of the knee: a comparison of hylan G-F 20 and a lower-molecular-weight hyaluronan. Clin Ther. 1999;21(9):1549–62.
92. Kotevoglu N, Iyibozkurt PC, Hiz O, et al. A prospective randomised controlled clinical trial comparing the efficacy of different molecular weight hyaluronan solutions in the treatment of knee osteoarthritis. Rheumatol Int. 2006;26(4):325–30.
93. Ghosh P, Guidolin D. Potential mechanism of action of intra-articular hyaluronan therapy in osteoarthritis: are the effects molecular weight dependent? Semin Arthritis Rheum. 2002;32(1):10–37.
94. Modawal A, Ferrer M, Choi HK, et al. Hyaluronic acid injections relieve knee pain. J Fam Pract. 2005;54(9):758–67.
95. Medina JM, Thomas A, Denegar CR. Knee osteoarthritis: should your patient opt for hyaluronic acid injection? J Fam Pract. 2006;55(8):669–75.
96. Campbell J, Bellamy N, Gee T. Differences between systematic reviews/meta-analyses of hyaluronic acid/hyaluronan/hylan in osteoarthritis of the knee. Osteoarthr Cartil. 2007;15(12):1424–36.
97. Tang SF, Chen CP, Chen MJ, et al. Changes in sagittal ground reaction forces after intra-articular hyaluronate injections for knee osteoarthritis. Arch Phys Med Rehabil. 2004;85(6):951–5.
98. Zoboli AA, de Rezende MU, de Campos GC, et al. Prospective randomized clinical trial: single and weekly viscosupplementation. Acta Ortop Bras. 2013;21(5):271–5.
99. Altman RD, Schemitsch E, Bedi A. Assessment of clinical practice guideline methodology for the treatment of knee osteoarthritis with intra-articular hyaluronic acid. Semin Arthritis Rheum. 2015;45:132.
100. Strand V, McIntyre LF, Beach WR, et al. Safety and efficacy of US-approved viscosupplements for knee osteoarthritis: a systematic review and meta-analysis of randomized, saline-controlled trials. J Pain Res. 2015;8:217–28.
101. Goldberg VM, Coutts RD. Pseudoseptic reactions to hylan viscosupplementation: diagnosis and treatment. Clin Orthop Relat Res. 2004;419:130–7.
102. Zhu Y, Yuan M, Meng HY, et al. Basic science and clinical application of platelet-rich plasma for cartilage defects and osteoarthritis: a review. Osteoarthr Cartil. 2013;21(11): 1627–37.
103. Riboh JC, Saltzman BM, Yanke AB, et al. Effect of leukocyte concentration on the efficacy of platelet-rich plasma in the treatment of knee osteoarthritis. Am J Sports Med. 2016;44(3):792–800.
104. Sanchez M, Anitua E, Azofra J, et al. Intra-articular injection of an autologous preparation rich in growth factors for the treatment of knee OA: a retrospective cohort study. Clin Exp Rheumatol. 2008;26(5):910–3.
105. Spakova T, Rosocha J, Lacko M, et al. Treatment of knee joint osteoarthritis with autologous platelet-rich plasma in comparison with hyaluronic acid. Am J Phys Med Rehabil. 2012;91(4):411–7.
106. Gobbi A, Lad D, Karnatzikos G. The effects of repeated intra-articular PRP injections on clinical outcomes of early osteoarthritis of the knee. Knee Surg Sports Traumatol Arthrosc. 2015;23(8):2170–7.
107. Filardo G, Kon E, Di Martino A, et al. Platelet-rich plasma vs hyaluronic acid to treat knee degenerative pathology: study design and preliminary results of a randomized controlled trial. BMC Musculoskelet Disord. 2012;13:229.
108. Filardo G, Di Matteo B, Di Martino A, et al. Platelet-rich plasma intra-articular knee injections show no superiority versus viscosupplementation: a randomized controlled trial. Am J Sports Med. 2015;43(7):1575–82.

109. Chang KV, Hung CY, Aliwarga F, et al. Comparative effectiveness of platelet-rich plasma injections for treating knee joint cartilage degenerative pathology: a systematic review and meta-analysis. Arch Phys Med Rehabil. 2014;95(3):562–75.
110. Campbell KA, Saltzman BM, Mascarenhas R, et al. Does intra-articular platelet-rich plasma injection provide clinically superior outcomes compared with other therapies in the treatment of knee osteoarthritis? A systematic review of overlapping meta-analyses. Arthroscopy. 2015;31(11):2213–21.
111. Oh JH, Kim W, Park KU, et al. Comparison of the cellular composition and cytokine-release kinetics of various platelet-rich plasma preparations. Am J Sports Med. 2015;43(12):3062–70.
112. Sakata R, McNary SM, Miyatake K, et al. Stimulation of the superficial zone protein and lubrication in the articular cartilage by human platelet-rich plasma. Am J Sports Med. 2015;43(6):1467–73.
113. Mishra AK, Skrepnik NV, Edwards SG, et al. Efficacy of platelet-rich plasma for chronic tennis elbow: a double-blind, prospective, multicenter, randomized controlled trial of 230 patients. Am J Sports Med. 2014;42(2):463–71.
114. Ornetti P, Nourissat G, Berenbaum F, et al. Does platelet-rich plasma have a role in the treatment of osteoarthritis? Joint Bone Spine. 2016;83(1):31–6.
115. Lee WD, Hurtig MB, Pilliar RM, et al. Engineering of hyaline cartilage with a calcified zone using bone marrow stromal cells. Osteoarthr Cartil. 2015;23(8):1307–15.
116. Qi Y, Feng G, Yan W. Mesenchymal stem cell-based treatment for cartilage defects in osteoarthritis. Mol Biol Rep. 2012;39(5):5683–9.
117. Matsumoto T, Cooper GM, Gharaibeh B, et al. Cartilage repair in a rat model of osteoarthritis through intraarticular transplantation of muscle-derived stem cells expressing bone morphogenetic protein 4 and soluble Flt-1. Arthritis Rheum. 2009;60(5):1390–405.
118. Gibbs N, Diamond R, Sekyere EO, et al. Management of knee osteoarthritis by combined stromal vascular fraction cell therapy, platelet-rich plasma, and musculoskeletal exercises: a case series. J Pain Res. 2015;8:799–806.
119. Vega A, Martin-Ferrero MA, Del Canto F, et al. Treatment of knee osteoarthritis with allogeneic bone marrow mesenchymal stem cells: a randomized controlled trial. Transplantation. 2015;99(8):1681–90.
120. Rodriguez-Merchan EC. Intra-articular injections of mesenchymal stem cells for knee osteoarthritis. Am J Orthop (Belle Mead NJ). 2014;43(12):E282–91.

Part II
Common Injuries in Masters Athletes, Treatment Considerations, and Return to Sports

Chapter 8
Knee Injuries: Conservative Management, Operative Management, and Return to Sport

Nicole A. Friel, Drew A. Lansdown, and Brian J. Cole

Introduction

Physical activity and participation in sports are increasing in all age groups, including masters athletes. The benefits of exercise range from physical to mental, and keeping the aging athlete healthy and active involves a multidisciplinary approach. Knee injuries are among the most common across all age groups, especially masters athletes. Acute injuries such as anterior cruciate ligament (ACL) tear and meniscus tear can occur in this population, yet knee osteoarthritis is the most prevalent musculoskeletal disease of the masters athlete [1].

ACL Injury

Injury to the anterior cruciate ligament is common in the active population. Young, active patients usually proceed to ACL reconstruction to restore the stability of the knee and return to activity. Treatment in older individuals is more controversial and may depend more upon the presence of demonstrative functional instability during desired activities. Many orthopedic surgeons choose to recommend prolonged non-operative treatment, citing surgery-related complications such as arthrofibrosis and decreased range of motion following surgery. However, several studies support the benefits of ACL reconstruction in older individuals, which are similar to their younger, active counterparts.

N. A. Friel, MD/MS · D. A. Lansdown, MD
Rush University Medical Center, Chicago, IL, USA

B. J. Cole, MD, MBA (✉)
Departments of Orthopedics and Surgery, Rush OPH, Shoulder, Elbow and Knee Surgery, Cartilage Restoration Center at Rush, Rush University Medical Center, Chicago, IL, USA
e-mail: bcole@rushortho.com

© Springer International Publishing AG, part of Springer Nature 2018
V. J. Wright, K. K. Middleton (eds.), *Masterful Care of the Aging Athlete*,
https://doi.org/10.1007/978-3-319-16223-2_8

The decision regarding non-operative versus operative treatment for ACL injury should be determined on an individual basis. Non-operative treatment may be appropriate for patients willing to refrain from sports or activities that require cutting, pivoting, and more acute directional changes. In athletes who participate in primarily straight-line activities, a normally functioning ACL may not be required or considered instrumental to these activities. Early rehabilitation to regain range of motion after injury is instrumental followed by strengthening exercises to maintain the stability of the joint even without an ACL.

In patients who participate in sports that involve directional change, persistent instability with conservative treatment may not be acceptable. ACL reconstruction decreases instability, and multiple studies in patients over 40 years show that patients have satisfactory outcomes. A systematic review by Mall et al. [2] concluded that ACL reconstruction can lead to excellent outcomes in patients older than 40 years who wish to maintain an active lifestyle or who otherwise have symptomatic instability with daily activities. Baker et al. [3] reviewed the results of 15 patients over the age of 60 at the time of ACL reconstruction. Thirteen of the 15 patients returned to sport or exercise, with one having undergone revision to total knee arthroplasty and the other deceased at the time of follow-up. It should be noted that preoperative radiographs showed no obvious evidence of arthritis in 10 (77%) patients and small osteophytes without loss of joint space were seen in 3 (23%) patients.

An ideal candidate for ACL reconstruction is someone without significant knee osteoarthritis. While ACL reconstruction can be pursued in those with osteoarthritis changes, some argue that patients will have unsuccessful outcomes due to the underling arthritis. Clearly, primary complaints of new-onset instability following an ACL tear without significant symptoms due to their underlying osteoarthritis can benefit from the stability provided by an ACL reconstruction. Concomitant procedures, such as osteotomy and cartilage restoration, can be considered in these cases with relevant arthritic change with or without malalignment. Further discussion regarding these treatment options is discussed below.

Knee Osteoarthritis

Arthritis is a highly prevalent condition that is estimated to affect 1 in 7 adults over their lifetime and 27–49.9 million adults in the United States alone [1, 4, 5]. Epidemiology studies estimate a lifetime risk of 45% for developing symptomatic knee osteoarthritis [6]. With an increasingly aging population, arthritis is expected to become both more prevalent and more impactful on patient quality of life [7]. There are numerous options, including conservative and surgical treatments for managing arthritis in the aging athlete to maintain activity levels and performance.

Conservative Treatment Options

Maintaining a healthy body weight is one recommendation that can limit aggravation of lower-extremity arthritis symptoms. The risk of developing symptomatic knee arthritis is doubled in obese patients relative to a patient with a normal BMI [8]. An increased body mass is the most important factor that contributes to an increased knee adductor moment, which has been linked to progression of symptomatic knee osteoarthritis [9]. Aaboe et al. demonstrated that losing weight can provide at least excellent short-term improvements in functional limitations by limiting joint loading in the setting of knee osteoarthritis [10].

Physical therapy can improve pain, function, and patient satisfaction in patients with osteoarthritis [11]. Deyle et al. reported that patients reported 20–40% relief in symptoms following only 2–3 treatments of exercise and manual therapy [12]. Targeted functional exercises have also shown benefit in the setting of knee osteoarthritis [13]. Importantly, muscular weakness has been correlated to range of motion in patients with knee arthritis, emphasizing the role of maintaining range of motion to preserve muscle function [14]. Aerobic exercises and strengthening exercises both lead to significant improvements in pain and function with adherence to these programs linked to improved outcomes [15–20].

Bracing may be an effective solution, especially for unicompartmental knee osteoarthritis. Raja et al. reported in a randomized control trial that a functional unloader brace significantly decreased pain relative to a simple neoprene sleeve for both flat walking and stair-climb tests [21]. Compliance with braces, however, is often an issue with only 25–41% of patients wearing a brace at 2 years after fitting [22, 23]. Additionally, a patient's financial responsibility for a functional brace can exceed $1500 [23].

Dietary supplements, especially glucosamine and chondroitin, are also frequently utilized in the setting of osteoarthritis. Glucosamine and chondroitin may have a role in increasing proteoglycan synthesis in cartilage [24, 25]. The commercial formulations, however, are highly variable and may not be consistent with contents described on labels [26, 27]. McAlindon et al. performed a meta-analysis of 15 placebo-controlled trials of glucosamine and/or chondroitin for patients with arthritis [28]. There was a moderate treatment effect for glucosamine and large treatment effect for chondroitin. These supplements may have a role in managing osteoarthritis, but inconsistencies in formulation may limit their effectiveness and utilization in clinical practice.

Nonsteroidal anti-inflammatory drugs (NSAIDs) are commonly prescribed for symptomatic management of arthritis with 65% of patients in the USA receiving these medications [29]. Da Costa et al. performed a meta-analysis of 74 randomized control trials that tested the efficacy of 7 NSAIDs and paracetamol (acetaminophen) for osteoarthritis of the knee and hip [30]. All medications provided demonstrable improvement in pain symptoms relative to placebo treatment. This study showed that diclofenac 150 mg per day showed the greatest effect for both pain and physical function. Despite their widespread use and proven effectiveness, NSAIDs do have potential systemic side effects. Diclofenac may increase the risk of cardiovascular complications, and naproxen increases the risk of upper gastrointestinal complications [30–32]. These side effects especially must be considered in the aging athlete with potential medical comorbidities [33].

Intra-articular injections are effective treatments that can minimize the risk of systemic complications. Corticosteroids are frequently administered and work to decrease the low-grade inflammation that is present during phases of osteoarthritis [34]. A systematic review of 27 trials of corticosteroids compared to control interventions showed moderate positive improvements at 1–2 weeks after injection, with small-to-moderate benefits noted at 4–6 weeks after injection [35]. There was no effect observed at 26 weeks after injection, suggesting that steroid injections confer a brief positive treatment effect.

Hyaluronic acid (HA) injections function by both mechanical viscosupplementation and by stimulating endogenous production of normal HA [36, 37]. These injections are only approved currently for use in the knee but do show significant improvements in symptomatic relief for greater duration than corticosteroid injections [38]. HA injections are offered in a variety of different formulations, though higher-molecular-weight formulations are more effective than low molecular weight [39]. Bannuru et al. showed intra-articular HA injections to be no different from continuous oral NSAIDs at 12 weeks after initiation of treatment, though HA injections did minimize the risk of potential NSAID-related side effects [40]. Intra-articular HA is administered in various numbers of injections and cycles, ranging from a single injection to five injections over four cycles [41]. An increasing number of injections may elevate the risk for potential adverse events [42].

Advances in biologic injections offer potential improvements in the conservative management of osteoarthritis. Platelet-rich plasma (PRP) is prepared from autologous venous blood and contains concentrated growth factors [43]. In vitro studies have demonstrated that PRP may help in cellular proliferation, collagen synthesis, and angiogenesis, and animal models have shown that PRP can reduce chondrolysis [43–46]. In vivo studies to date have mixed results on the benefit in the setting of osteoarthritis. Sampson et al. reported that three PRP injections for symptomatic knee arthritis produced significant improvement in KOOS scores, pain, and function at 12 weeks after injection. Compared to corticosteroid injections, a randomized control trial concludes that PRP decreased pain at a greater magnitude and for longer duration than corticosteroid alone and improved quality of life [47]. Studies that have compared PRP to HA show mixed results. A randomized controlled trial showed no difference between the two with an increase in postinjection swelling and pain observed in the PRP group [48, 49]. However, another study reviewing three meta-analyses found significant improvements in patient outcomes at both 6 and 12 months postinjection when comparing intra-articular PRP injection to either intra-articular HA or placebo injection [50]. There can be great variability with regard to PRP content and effectiveness, and further studies are needed to better define the role of this treatment in routine clinical practice [43, 51]. Mesenchymal stem cell injections may also improve symptoms for patients with osteoarthritis, likely due to their immunosuppressive and anti-inflammatory activities [52]. In a controlled trial of bone marrow aspirate concentrate versus saline injections, Shapiro et al. demonstrated that intra-articular BMAC injections are safe, though pain improved at similar levels for both treatment arms up to 6 months after injection [53]. Additional further research on stem cell treatments will elucidate the role these injections may have for management of osteoarthritis [10].

Surgical Treatment Options

Cartilage regeneration can play a role in the surgical management for patients with focal cartilage defects. Biological treatments for focal chondral lesions such as debridement, abrasion, microfracture, osteochondral autograft or allograft, and various other cell-based strategies have shown good results in young patients [44]. As patients age, they are less likely to have the small, acute, focal defects that respond well to cartilage restoration. However, age is not an absolute contraindication to cartilage restoration. Surgical decision-making may vary from patient to patient based on patient age, defect-related surgical history, lesion size, opposing articular surfaces, meniscal function, mechanical alignment, ligament instability, body mass index, and recovery expectations [54]. Microfracture is a first-line treatment option for focal cartilage defects, with a high rate of success in returning athletes to demanding, high-impact sports participation [55]. The authors note, however, that better outcomes are seen in patients who are younger and have a smaller defect size, short duration of symptoms, fewer prior surgical interventions, and better repair cartilage morphology. Similarly, favorable outcomes are reported for osteochondral allograft transplantation, in which patients with osteochondritis dissecans and traumatic and idiopathic etiologies have more favorable outcomes, as do younger patients with unipolar lesions and short symptom duration [56]. In a review of cartilage restoration procedures of the knee, Bedi et al. remind readers that while bone marrow stimulation procedures and whole-tissue transplantation of allografts or autografts can achieve favorable outcomes, they are not without complications [57]. Concomitant procedures must address instability, alignment, and meniscal deficiency, if necessary. Therefore, patient selection remains critical for masters athletes with focal cartilage lesions.

Large, non-focal cartilage damage affecting an entire compartment of the knee can often be treated with one of two surgical procedures: high tibial osteotomy or unicompartmental knee replacement. For medial tibiofemoral arthritis, a HTO moves the mechanical axis of the lower limb laterally to redistribute the weight-bearing forces away from the involved medial compartment. Patients who have undergone HTO have improvement in their pain and are able to increase their activity level postoperatively [58–61]. Patients return to a number of sports, including demanding sports such as downhill skiing and mountain biking [62].

High tibial osteotomy is generally indicated for young, active, nonobese patients with isolated medial tibiofemoral arthritis, good knee stability, and preserved range of motion. In a study to assess preoperative predictors of survival and functional outcome with a lateral closing-wedge HTO, Howells et al. [63] showed that improved survival is associated with age <55 years, preoperative WOMAC scores >45, and a BMI <30. However, the authors also show that in patients over 55 years of age with adequate preoperative functional scores, survival can be good and functional outcomes can be significantly better than their younger counterparts. Bonnin et al. [59] reported on outcomes after HTO and sought to determine how patient expectations and motivation relate to outcome. There was a strong correlation between activity participation and motivation, with young motivated patients returning to strenuous activities following HTO.

Unicompartmental knee arthroplasty is another option to treat patients with arthritic changes affecting one compartment. For medial tibiofemoral arthritis, indications are similar to that for HTO, in which appropriate patients include those who are nonobese with unicompartmental arthritis, well-preserved joint alignment, ligamentous stability, and well-preserved range of motion. Outcomes of UKA are generally very good with most recent studies showing implant survivorship over 80% at a minimum of 10-year follow-up [64–68].

There is considerable overlap in the indications for HTO and UKA. Yim et al. [69] identified no significant differences between HTO and UKA for medial unicompartmental osteoarthritis in terms of return to recreational activity including cycling, swimming, exercise walking, jogging, dancing, and mountain climbing and short-term clinical outcomes. In a meta-analysis, Spahn et al. [70] found that there were no differences in the clinical outcomes for patients undergoing HTO or UKA, but suggested that HTO is more appropriate for younger patients who accept a slight decrease in their physical activity, while medial UKA is appropriate for older patients obtaining sufficient pain relief but with reduced physical activity. Despite similar clinical outcomes, there is an increasing utilization of UKA and a declining utilization of HTO when performed for the management of unicompartmental osteoarthritis. However, HTOs are still seen as an important procedure in young males with medial compartmental arthritis [71].

Much less common than medial compartment arthritis is isolated lateral compartment or isolated patellofemoral arthritis. Similar to medial compartment arthritis, surgical options for isolated lateral tibiofemoral arthritis include osteotomy, including distal femoral and high tibial, as well as unicompartmental knee arthroplasty. The literature is varus osteotomies for lateral compartment disease is sparse, but 10-year cumulative survival rates of 64–90% are reported [72–74]. Lateral UKA outcomes are favorable, with several authors reporting survivorship over 90% [72, 75, 76]; however, there is little discussion regarding return to activity. Patients with isolated patellofemoral disease are managed conservatively for extended periods of time, and operative treatment is only considered when all non-operative means are completely exhausted. In select patients with large patellofemoral chondral defects and intractable anterior knee pain, patellofemoral arthroplasty can be performed.

Arthroplasty, whether with a UKA or a total knee arthroplasty (TKA), offers a reliable treatment option for patients with osteoarthritic changes; however, there is concern regarding the survival of the prosthesis in active patients who place greater demands on their knee [77, 78]. Compared with patients with a low activity level after arthroplasty, patients who participate in athletic activity have increased force crossing the reconstructed joint, increased joint-bearing-surface wear, increased stress at the bone-implant fixation surface, and a higher prevalence of traumatic injury to the joint [77, 79, 80]. However, there is no consensus regarding recommendations and restrictions of activity following arthroplasty. In general, orthopedic surgeons allow low-impact activities such as golf, swimming, and cycling but recommend against high-impact activities such as basketball, jogging, and soccer [77]. Importantly, patients should be encouraged to resume activity based upon the cardiovascular and mental benefits as well as their enjoyment of activity, but also with an education of the risks associated with specific activity and an understanding of the importance of stretching and strengthening to reduce problems.

Summary

Knee injuries in masters athletes range from acute injuries such as ACL tears to degenerative changes leading to osteoarthritis. Appropriate treatment allows the athlete to return to the physical and mental benefits of exercise. Acute knee injuries such as ACL tears can be treated non-operatively with physical therapy in a select group of patients, but high-demand athletes involved in activities with directional change benefit from ACL reconstruction. Knee osteoarthritis is addressed with a progression of treatment options, including maintenance of a healthy weight, physical therapy, bracing, oral supplements, NSAIDs, and varying intra-articular injections, including corticosteroid, hyaluronic acid, and biologic injections. Surgical treatments include cartilage restoration, osteotomy, and partial or total knee arthroplasty. The ultimate goal is to increase function and decrease pain to allow the masters athlete return to activity.

References

1. Lawrence RC, Felson DT, Helmick CG, Arnold LM, Choi H, Deyo RA, Gabriel S, Hirsch R, Hochberg MC, Hunder GG, Jordan JM, Katz JN, Kremers HM, Wolfe F, National Arthritis Data Workgroup. Estimates of the prevalence of arthritis and other rheumatic conditions in the United States: Part II. Arthritis Rheum. 2008;58(1):26–35. https://doi.org/10.1002/art.23176.
2. Mall NA, Frank RM, Saltzman BM, Cole BJ, Bach BR Jr. Results after anterior cruciate ligament reconstruction in patients older than 40 years: how do they compare with younger patients? A systematic review and comparison with younger populations. Sports Health. 2016;8(2):177–81. https://doi.org/10.1177/1941738115622138.
3. Baker CL Jr, Jones JC, Zhang J. Long-term outcomes after anterior cruciate ligament reconstruction in patients 60 years and older. Orthop J Sports Med. 2014;2(12):2325967114561737. https://doi.org/10.1177/2325967114561737.

4. Cheng Y, Hootman J, Murphy L, Langmaid G, Helmich C. Prevalence of doctor-diagnosed arthritis and arthritis-attributable activity limitation-United States, 2007-2009. Morb Mortal Wkly Rep. 2010;59(39):1261–5.
5. Losina E, Weinstein AM, Reichmann WM, Burbine SA, Solomon DH, Daigle ME, Rome BN, Chen SP, Hunter DJ, Suter LG. Lifetime risk and age at diagnosis of symptomatic knee osteo-arthritis in the US. Arthritis Care Res. 2013;65(5):703–11.
6. Jordan JM, Helmick CG, Renner JB, Luta G, Dragomir AD, Woodard J, Fang F, Schwartz TA, Abbate LM, Callahan LF. Prevalence of knee symptoms and radiographic and symptomatic knee osteoarthritis in African Americans and Caucasians: the Johnston County Osteoarthritis Project. J Rheumatol. 2007;34(1):172–80.
7. Bernstein A, Hing E, Moss A, Allen K, Siller A, Tiggle R. Health care in America: trends in utilization. Hyattsville: National Center for Health Statistics; 2003.
8. Murphy L, Schwartz TA, Helmick CG, Renner JB, Tudor G, Koch G, Dragomir A, Kalsbeek WD, Luta G, Jordan JM. Lifetime risk of symptomatic knee osteoarthritis. Arthritis Care Res. 2008;59(9):1207–13. https://doi.org/10.1002/art.24021.
9. Adams T, Band-Entrup D, Kuhn S, Legere L, Mace K, Paggi A, Penney M. Physical ther-apy management of knee osteoarthritis in the middle-aged athlete. Sports Med Arthrosc Rev. 2013;21(1):2–10.
10. Aaboe J, Bliddal H, Messier S, Alkjaer T, Henriksen M. Effects of an intensive weight loss program on knee joint loading in obese adults with knee osteoarthritis. Osteoarthr Cartil. 2011;19(7):822–8.
11. Pollard H, Ward G, Hoskins W, Hardy K. The effect of a manual therapy knee protocol on osteoarthritic knee pain: a randomised controlled trial. J Can Chiropr Assoc. 2008;52(4):229.
12. Deyle GD, Allison SC, Matekel RL, Ryder MG, Stang JM, Gohdes DD, Hutton JP, Henderson NE, Garber MB. Physical therapy treatment effectiveness for osteoarthritis of the knee: a ran-domized comparison of supervised clinical exercise and manual therapy procedures versus a home exercise program. Phys Ther. 2005;85(12):1301–17.
13. Farr JN, Going SB, McKnight PE, Kasle S, Cussler EC, Cornett M. Progressive resistance training improves overall physical activity levels in patients with early osteoarthritis of the knee: a randomized controlled trial. Phys Ther. 2010;90(3):356–66.
14. Weng M-C, Lee C-L, Chen C-H, Hsu J-J, Lee W-D, Huang M-H, Chen T-W. Effects of differ-ent stretching techniques on the outcomes of isokinetic exercise in patients with knee osteoar-thritis. Kaohsiung J Med Sci. 2009;25(6):306–15.
15. Patrick DL, Ramsey SD, Spencer AC, Kinne S, Belza B, Topolski TD. Economic evaluation of aquatic exercise for persons with osteoarthritis. Med Care. 2001;39(5):413–24.
16. Penninx BW, Messier SP, Rejeski WJ, Williamson JD, DiBari M, Cavazzini C, Applegate WB, Pahor M. Physical exercise and the prevention of disability in activities of daily living in older persons with osteoarthritis. Arch Intern Med. 2001;161(19):2309–16.
17. Penninx BW, Rejeski WJ, Pandya J, Miller ME, Di Bari M, Applegate WB, Pahor M. Exercise and depressive symptoms a comparison of aerobic and resistance exercise effects on emo-tional and physical function in older persons with high and low depressive symptomatology. J Gerontol Ser B Psychol Sci Soc Sci. 2002;57(2):P124–32.
18. Rejeski WJ, Brawley LR, Ettinger W, Morgan T, Thompson C. Compliance to exercise ther-apy in older participants with knee osteoarthritis: implications for treating disability. Med Sci Sports Exerc. 1997;29(8):977–85.
19. Shamliyan TA, Wang S-Y, Olson-Kellogg B, Kane RL. Physical therapy interventions for knee pain secondary to osteoarthritis: a systematic review. Ann Intern Med. 2012;157(9):632–44.
20. van Gool CH, Penninx BW, Kempen GI, Rejeski WJ, Miller GD, van Eijk JTM, Pahor M, Messier SP. Effects of exercise adherence on physical function among overweight older adults with knee osteoarthritis. Arthritis Care Res. 2005;53(1):24–32.
21. Raja K, Dewan N. Efficacy of knee braces and foot orthoses in conservative management of knee osteoarthritis: a systematic review. Am J Phys Med Rehabil. 2011;90(3):247–62. https://doi.org/10.1097/PHM.0b013e318206386b.

22. Barnes CL, Cawley PW, Hederman B. Effect of CounterForce brace on symptomatic relief in a group of patients with symptomatic unicompartmental osteoarthritis: a prospective 2-year investigation. Am J Orthop (Belle Mead NJ). 2002;31(7):396–401.
23. Squyer E, Stamper DL, Hamilton DT, Sabin JA, Leopold SS. Unloader knee braces for osteoarthritis: do patients actually wear them? Clin Orthop Relat Res. 2013;471(6):1982–91.
24. Bassleer C, Rovati L, Franchimont P. Stimulation of proteoglycan production by glucosamine sulfate in chondrocytes isolated from human osteoarthritic articular cartilage in vitro. Osteoarthr Cartil. 1998;6(6):427–34.
25. Uebelhart D, Thonar EJA, Zhang J, Williams JM. Protective effect of exogenous chondroitin 4, 6-sulfate in the acute degradation of articular cartilage in the rabbit. Osteoarthr Cartil. 1998;6:6–13.
26. Adebowale AO, Cox DS, Liang Z, Eddington ND. Analysis of glucosamine and chondroitin sulfate content in marketed products and the Caco-2 permeability of chondroitin sulfate raw materials. J Am Nutrac Assoc. 2000;3(1):37–44.
27. Russell AS, Aghazadeh-Habashi A, Jamali F. Active ingredient consistency of commercially available glucosamine sulfate products. J Rheumatol. 2002;29(11):2407–9.
28. McAlindon TE, LaValley MP, Gulin JP, Felson DT. Glucosamine and chondroitin for treatment of osteoarthritis: a systematic quality assessment and meta-analysis. JAMA. 2000;283(11):1469–75.
29. Gore M, Tai KS, Sadosky A, Leslie D, Stacey BR. Use and costs of prescription medications and alternative treatments in patients with osteoarthritis and chronic low back pain in community-based settings. Pain Pract. 2012;12(7):550–60.
30. da Costa BR, Reichenbach S, Keller N, Nartey L, Wandel S, Jüni P, Trelle S. Effectiveness of non-steroidal anti-inflammatory drugs for the treatment of pain in knee and hip osteoarthritis: a network meta-analysis. Lancet. 2016;387(10033):2093–105. https://doi.org/10.1016/s0140-6736(16)30002-2.
31. Bhala N, Emberson J, Merhi A, Abramson S, Arber N, Baron J, Bombardier C, Cannon C, Farkouh M, FitzGerald G. Vascular and upper gastrointestinal effects of non-steroidal anti-inflammatory drugs: meta-analyses of individual participant data from randomised trials. Lancet. 2013;382(9894):769–79.
32. Trelle S, Reichenbach S, Wandel S, Hildebrand P, Tschannen B, Villiger PM, Egger M, Jüni P. Cardiovascular safety of non-steroidal anti-inflammatory drugs: network meta-analysis. BMJ. 2011;342:c7086.
33. Roberts E, Nunes VD, Buckner S, Latchem S, Constanti M, Miller P, Doherty M, Zhang W, Birrell F, Porcheret M. Paracetamol: not as safe as we thought? A systematic literature review of observational studies. Ann Rheum Dis. 2016;75(3):552–9.
34. Creamer P. Intra-articular corticosteroid injections in osteoarthritis: do they work and if so, how? Ann Rheum Dis. 1997;56(11):634–5.
35. Jüni P, Hari R, Rutjes AW, Fischer R, Silletta MG, Reichenbach S, da Costa BR. Intra-articular corticosteroid for knee osteoarthritis. Cochrane Database Syst Rev. 2015;(10):CD005328.
36. Hochberg MC, Altman RD, April KT, Benkhalti M, Guyatt G, McGowan J, Towheed T, Welch V, Wells G, Tugwell P. American College of Rheumatology 2012 recommendations for the use of nonpharmacologic and pharmacologic therapies in osteoarthritis of the hand, hip, and knee. Arthritis Care Res. 2012;64(4):465–74.
37. McAlindon TE, Bannuru RR, Sullivan MC, Arden NK, Berenbaum F, Bierma-Zeinstra SM, Hawker GA, Henrotin Y, Hunter DJ, Kawaguchi H, Kwoh K, Lohmander S, Rannou F, Roos EM, Underwood M. OARSI guidelines for the non-surgical management of knee osteoarthritis. Osteoarthr Cartil. 2014;22(3):363–88. https://doi.org/10.1016/j.joca.2014.01.003.
38. Bannuru RR, Natov NS, Dasi UR, Schmid CH, McAlindon TE. Therapeutic trajectory following intra-articular hyaluronic acid injection in knee osteoarthritis--meta-analysis. Osteoarthr Cartil. 2011;19(6):611–9. https://doi.org/10.1016/j.joca.2010.09.014.
39. Lo GH, LaValley M, McAlindon T, Felson DT. Intra-articular hyaluronic acid in treatment of knee osteoarthritis: a meta-analysis. JAMA. 2003;290(23):3115–21.

40. Bannuru RR, Vaysbrot EE, Sullivan MC, McAlindon TE. Relative efficacy of hyaluronic acid in comparison with NSAIDs for knee osteoarthritis: a systematic review and meta-analysis. Semin Arthritis Rheum. 2014;43(5):593–9. https://doi.org/10.1016/j.semarthrit.2013.10.002.

41. Richette P, Chevalier X, Ea HK, Eymard F, Henrotin Y, Ornetti P, Sellam J, Cucherat M, Marty M. Hyaluronan for knee osteoarthritis: an updated meta-analysis of trials with low risk of bias. RMD open. 2015;1(1):e000071.

42. Rutjes AW, Jüni P, da Costa BR, Trelle S, Nüesch E, Reichenbach S. Viscosupplementation for osteoarthritis of the knee: a systematic review and meta-analysis. Ann Intern Med. 2012;157(3):180–91.

43. Pintan GF, de Oliveira AS Jr, Lenza M, Antonioli E, Ferretti M. Update on biological therapies for knee injuries: osteoarthritis. Curr Rev Muscoskelet Med. 2014;7(3):263–9.

44. Filardo G, Kon E, Andriolo L, Di Matteo B, Balboni F, Marcacci M. Clinical profiling in cartilage regeneration: prognostic factors for midterm results of matrix-assisted autologous chondrocyte transplantation. Am J Sports Med. 2014;42(4):898–905. https://doi.org/10.1177/0363546513518552.

45. Koh YG, Choi YJ, Kwon SK, Kim YS, Yeo JE. Clinical results and second-look arthroscopic findings after treatment with adipose-derived stem cells for knee osteoarthritis. Knee Surg Sports Traumatol Arthrosc. 2015;23(5):1308–16. https://doi.org/10.1007/s00167-013-2807-2.

46. Saito M, Takahashi K, Arai E, Inoue A, Sakao K, Tonomura H, Honjo K, Nakagawa S, Inoue H, Tabata Y. Intra-articular administration of platelet-rich plasma with biodegradable gelatin hydrogel microspheres prevents osteoarthritis progression in the rabbit knee. Clin Exp Rheumatol. 2009;27(2):201.

47. Forogh B, Mianehsaz E, Shoaee S, Ahadi T, Raissi GR, Sajadi S. Effect of single injection of platelet-rich plasma in comparison with corticosteroid on knee osteoarthritis: a double-blind randomized clinical trial. J Sports Med Phys Fitness. 2016;56(7–8):901–8.

48. Filardo G, Di Matteo B, Di Martino A, Merli ML, Cenacchi A, Fornasari P, Marcacci M, Kon E. Platelet-rich plasma intra-articular knee injections show no superiority versus viscosupplementation a randomized controlled trial. Am J Sports Med. 2015;43(7):1575–82.

49. Görmeli G, Görmeli CA, Ataoglu B, Çolak C, Aslantürk O, Ertem K. Multiple PRP injections are more effective than single injections and hyaluronic acid in knees with early osteoarthritis: a randomized, double-blind, placebo-controlled trial. Knee Surg Sports Traumatol Arthrosc. 2015;25(3):958–65. https://doi.org/10.1007/s00167-015-3705-6.

50. Campbell KA, Saltzman BM, Mascarenhas R, Khair MM, Verma NN, Bach BR Jr, Cole BJ. Does intra-articular platelet-rich plasma injection provide clinically superior outcomes compared with other therapies in the treatment of knee osteoarthritis? A systematic review of overlapping meta-analyses. Arthroscopy. 2015;31(11):2213–21. https://doi.org/10.1016/j.arthro.2015.03.041.

51. Ornetti P, Nourissat G, Berenbaum F, Sellam J, Richette P, Chevalier X, under the aegis of the Osteoarthritis Section of the French Society for Rheumatology. Does platelet-rich plasma have a role in the treatment of osteoarthritis? Joint Bone Spine. 2016;83(1):31–6. https://doi.org/10.1016/j.jbspin.2015.05.002.

52. Beitzel K, McCarthy MB, Cote MP, Chowaniec D, Falcone LM, Falcone JA, Dugdale EM, DeBerardino TM, Arciero RA, Mazzocca AD. Rapid isolation of human stem cells (connective progenitor cells) from the distal femur during arthroscopic knee surgery. Arthroscopy. 2012;28(1):74–84.

53. Shapiro SA, Kazmerchak SE, Heckman MG, Zubair AC, O'Connor MI. A prospective, single-blind, placebo-controlled trial of bone marrow aspirate concentrate for knee osteoarthritis. Am J Sports Med. 2016;45(1):82–90. https://doi.org/10.1177/0363546516662455.

54. Pascual-Garrido C, Daley E, Verma NN, Cole BJ. A comparison of the outcomes for cartilage defects of the knee treated with biologic resurfacing versus focal metallic implants. Arthroscopy. 2016;33:364. https://doi.org/10.1016/j.arthro.2016.07.010.

55. Mithoefer K, Gill TJ, Cole BJ, Williams RJ, Mandelbaum BR. Clinical outcome and return to competition after microfracture in the Athlete's knee: an evidence-based systematic review. Cartilage. 2010;1(2):113–20. https://doi.org/10.1177/1947603510366576.
56. Chahal J, Gross AE, Gross C, Mall N, Dwyer T, Chahal A, Whelan DB, Cole BJ. Outcomes of osteochondral allograft transplantation in the knee. Arthroscopy. 2013;29(3):575–88. https://doi.org/10.1016/j.arthro.2012.12.002.
57. Bedi A, Feeley BT, Williams RJ 3rd. Management of articular cartilage defects of the knee. J Bone Joint Surg Am. 2010;92(4):994–1009. https://doi.org/10.2106/JBJS.I.00895.
58. Akizuki S, Shibakawa A, Takizawa T, Yamazaki I, Horiuchi H. The long-term outcome of high tibial osteotomy: a ten- to 20-year follow-up. J Bone Joint Surg Br. 2008;90(5):592–6. https://doi.org/10.1302/0301-620X.90B5.20386.
59. Bonnin MP, Laurent JR, Zadegan F, Badet R, Pooler Archbold HA, Servien E. Can patients really participate in sport after high tibial osteotomy? Knee Surg Sports Traumatol Arthrosc. 2013;21(1):64–73. https://doi.org/10.1007/s00167-011-1461-9.
60. Hernigou P, Medevielle D, Debeyre J, Goutallier D. Proximal tibial osteotomy for osteoarthritis with varus deformity. A ten to thirteen-year follow-up study. J Bone Joint Surg Am. 1987;69(3):332–54.
61. Waterman BR, Hoffmann JD, Laughlin MD, Burks R, Pallis MP, Tokish JM, Belmont PJ Jr. Success of high tibial osteotomy in the United States Military. Orthop J Sports Med. 2015;3(3):2325967115574670. https://doi.org/10.1177/2325967115574670.
62. Salzmann GM, Ahrens P, Naal FD, El-Azab H, Spang JT, Imhoff AB, Lorenz S. Sporting activity after high tibial osteotomy for the treatment of medial compartment knee osteoarthritis. Am J Sports Med. 2009;37(2):312–8. https://doi.org/10.1177/0363546508325666.
63. Howells NR, Salmon L, Waller A, Scanelli J, Pinczewski LA. The outcome at ten years of lateral closing-wedge high tibial osteotomy: determinants of survival and functional outcome. Bone Joint J. 2014;96-B(11):1491–7. https://doi.org/10.1302/0301-620X.96B11.33617.
64. Bonasia DE, Dettoni F, Sito G, Blonna D, Marmotti A, Bruzzone M, Castoldi F, Rossi R. Medial opening wedge high tibial osteotomy for medial compartment overload/arthritis in the varus knee: prognostic factors. Am J Sports Med. 2014;42(3):690–8. https://doi.org/10.1177/0363546513516577.
65. Foran JR, Brown NM, Della Valle CJ, Berger RA, Galante JO. Long-term survivorship and failure modes of unicompartmental knee arthroplasty. Clin Orthop Relat Res. 2013;471(1):102–8. https://doi.org/10.1007/s11999-012-2517-y.
66. O'Rourke MR, Gardner JJ, Callaghan JJ, Liu SS, Goetz DD, Vittetoe DA, Sullivan PM, Johnston RC. The John Insall Award: unicompartmental knee replacement: a minimum twenty-one-year followup, end-result study. Clin Orthop Relat Res. 2005;440:27–37.
67. Steele RG, Hutabarat S, Evans RL, Ackroyd CE, Newman JH. Survivorship of the St Georg Sled medial unicompartmental knee replacement beyond ten years. J Bone Joint Surg Br. 2006;88(9):1164–8. https://doi.org/10.1302/0301-620X.88B9.18044.
68. Svard UC, Price AJ. Oxford medial unicompartmental knee arthroplasty. A survival analysis of an independent series. J Bone Joint Surg Br. 2001;83(2):191–4.
69. Yim JH, Song EK, Seo HY, Kim MS, Seon JK. Comparison of high tibial osteotomy and unicompartmental knee arthroplasty at a minimum follow-up of 3 years. J Arthroplast. 2013;28(2):243–7. https://doi.org/10.1016/j.arth.2012.06.011.
70. Spahn G, Hofmann GO, von Engelhardt LV, Li M, Neubauer H, Klinger HM. The impact of a high tibial valgus osteotomy and unicondylar medial arthroplasty on the treatment for knee osteoarthritis: a meta-analysis. Knee Surg Sports Traumatol Arthrosc. 2013;21(1):96–112. https://doi.org/10.1007/s00167-011-1751-2.
71. Nwachukwu BU, McCormick FM, Schairer WW, Frank RM, Provencher MT, Roche MW. Unicompartmental knee arthroplasty versus high tibial osteotomy: United States practice patterns for the surgical treatment of unicompartmental arthritis. J Arthroplast. 2014;29(8):1586–9. https://doi.org/10.1016/j.arth.2014.04.002.

72. Scott CE, Nutton RW, Biant LC. Lateral compartment osteoarthritis of the knee: biomechanics and surgical management of end-stage disease. Bone Joint J. 2013;95-B(4):436–44. https://doi.org/10.1302/0301-620X.95B4.30536.

73. Sternheim A, Garbedian S, Backstein D. Distal femoral varus osteotomy: unloading the lateral compartment: long-term follow-up of 45 medial closing wedge osteotomies. Orthopedics. 2011;34(9):e488–90. https://doi.org/10.3928/01477447-20110714-37.

74. Wang JW, Hsu CC. Distal femoral varus osteotomy for osteoarthritis of the knee. J Bone Joint Surg Am. 2005;87(1):127–33. https://doi.org/10.2106/JBJS.C.01559.

75. Argenson JN, Parratte S, Bertani A, Flecher X, Aubaniac JM. Long-term results with a lateral unicondylar replacement. Clin Orthop Relat Res. 2008;466(11):2686–93. https://doi.org/10.1007/s11999-008-0351-z.

76. Lustig S, Elguindy A, Servien E, Fary C, Munini E, Demey G, Neyret P. 5- to 16-year follow-up of 54 consecutive lateral unicondylar knee arthroplasties with a fixed-all polyethylene bearing. J Arthroplast. 2011;26(8):1318–25. https://doi.org/10.1016/j.arth.2011.01.015.

77. Healy WL, Sharma S, Schwartz B, Iorio R. Athletic activity after total joint arthroplasty. J Bone Joint Surg Am. 2008;90(10):2245–52. https://doi.org/10.2106/JBJS.H.00274.

78. Parratte S, Argenson JN, Pearce O, Pauly V, Auquier P, Aubaniac JM. Medial unicompartmental knee replacement in the under-50s. J Bone Joint Surg Br. 2009;91(3):351–6. https://doi.org/10.1302/0301-620X.91B3.21588.

79. Lavernia CJ, Sierra RJ, Hungerford DS, Krackow K. Activity level and wear in total knee arthroplasty: a study of autopsy retrieved specimens. J Arthroplasty. 2001;16(4):446–53. https://doi.org/10.1054/arth.2001.23509.

80. Schmalzried TP, Shepherd EF, Dorey FJ, Jackson WO, dela Rosa M, Fa'vae F, McKellop HA, McClung CD, Martell J, Moreland JR, Amstutz HC. The John Charnley Award. Wear is a function of use, not time. Clin Orthop Relat Res. 2000;(381):36–46.

Chapter 9
Common Hip Injuries: Conservative Management

Vonda J. Wright, Philip Zakko, Edward Chang, and Kellie K. Middleton

Non-operative Hip Preservation

Master athletes participate in a wide range of sports including tennis, golf, running, and cycling. Each of these activities requires stability, flexibility, full range of motion (ROM), and efficient strength and power of core and hip muscles including the rectus abdominis, gluteal muscles or abductors, piriformis and external rotators, adductors, iliacus, and psoas muscles. Hip injuries can significantly hinder range of motion and stability, thus altering native hip biomechanics and preventing peak performance. While younger athletes (in their second and third decades) are more prone to acute apophyseal and epiphyseal injuries due to lack of ossification of their cartilaginous growth plates, older athletes are more susceptible to chronic injuries secondary to overuse and inflammation. Such pathologies include anterior and posterior adhesive capsulitis, greater trochanteric bursitis, piriformis syndrome, and stress fractures [1]. Degenerative changes of the hip can also be a major cause of hip pain in aging athletes.

V. J. Wright, MD, MS
Department of Orthopaedic Surgery, University of Pittsburgh,
UPMC Lemieux Sports Complex, Pittsburgh, PA, USA
e-mail: vonda.wright@northside.com

P. Zakko, BSA
University of Pittsburgh Medical Center, Farmington, CT, USA

E. Chang, MD
Inova Health System, Alexandria, VA, USA

K. K. Middleton, MD, MPH (✉)
Department of Orthopaedic Surgery,
University of Pittsburgh Medical Center, Pittsburgh, PA, USA
e-mail: middletonkk@upmc.edu

© Springer International Publishing AG, part of Springer Nature 2018   89
V. J. Wright, K. K. Middleton (eds.), *Masterful Care of the Aging Athlete*,
https://doi.org/10.1007/978-3-319-16223-2_9

Adhesive Capsulitis

Adhesive capsulitis of the hip (ACH) is most commonly seen in middle-aged individuals, making it especially concerning to master athletes. ACH is characterized by a painful decrease in active and passive ROM as synovial inflammation in the acute stages (stages 1–2) of the disease progresses to capsular fibrosis in the chronic stages (stages 3–4) [2]. Primary management of ACH should involve pharmacology and physical therapy in the acute stages, while surgical management can be incorporated into treatment in the chronic stages. Many case reports have indicated spontaneous resolution of ACH symptoms [3–6]; thus, more conservative management strategies are recommended.

Treatment of ACH in the acute stages should focus on reducing inflammation, addressing associated pathologies, and correcting underlying etiologies. Oral NSAIDs and intra-articular steroid and/or analgesic injections were found to be effective in managing the pain associated with ACH [7]. In addition to NSAIDS and injections, stage-based physical therapy regimens should be incorporated.

ACH appears to be more common than the literature suggests; thus, current physical therapy models are based on treatment models for adhesive capsulitis of the shoulder (ACS). The proposed pathophysiology of ACH is biomechanical dysfunction of the hip and/or related joints. As such, physical therapy programs should emphasize strength of core and associated hip muscles [8].

Greater Trochanteric Bursitis

Greater trochanteric bursitis is a commonly diagnosed inflammatory condition with pain localized at the greater trochanter that radiates down to the buttock and lateral aspect of the thigh. Its prevalence is most often found in middle-aged patients and is associated with overuse, trauma, or any conditions that may alter normal gait patterns [9]. Therefore, this condition is extremely relevant to the aging athlete.

On physical examination, patients often present with tenderness to palpation about the greater trochanter, lateral hip pain, pain on hip abduction against resistance, pain radiating down the lateral aspect of the affected lower extremity, a positive Patrick-FABERE (hip flexion, abduction, external rotation, and extension) test and often a positive Ober's test for iliotibial band tightness [10]. These symptoms are often effectively treated non-operatively with rest, ice, anti-inflammatory medications, and physical therapy. Both passive and active stretching, including neuromuscular facilitation techniques, and maintaining normal hip ROM are essential to a successful rehabilitation process. Furthermore, associated back, hip, or core strength abnormalities can often affect gait, resulting in bursitis [11]. Thus, assessment of gait is important for both diagnostic and treatment purposes. Patients presenting with antalgic gait should be evaluated for strength abnormalities by utilizing functional tests such as the single-leg squat and the thoracic spine evaluation.

An individualized (or patient-specific) physical therapy routine can then be recommended to target any weaknesses most specifically focused on gluteus medius and core strength and ITB tissue release via active tissue release or foam rolling.

When noninvasive conservative methods fail, local anesthetic and corticosteroid injections have been shown to provide effective pain relief of trochanteric bursitis in 60–100% of patients [12] PRP/ACP injections are quickly rising as a common adjunct to care for decreasing inflammatory and structural injury. Surgical treatment—often in the form of bursectomy—should be considered only if symptoms persist after 6 months of non-operative treatment [13].

Piriformis Syndrome

Piriformis syndrome (PS) is a neuromuscular disorder that results from the piriformis muscle compressing the sciatic nerve. The piriformis muscle is involved in stabilizing the hip joint, flexing and externally rotating the femur. Research suggests that gluteal trauma and posttraumatic scarring around the hip and gluteal regions are important causes of PS [14]. In addition, the piriformis muscle itself can spasm from hypertrophy and overuse are also possible etiologies [15]. PS is associated with low back pain, buttocks pain, and sciatica, with symptoms exacerbated by sitting.

Treatment for PS should begin conservatively. It is typical to administer various medications for neuropathic pain such as NSAIDs and muscle relaxants, concomitantly with physical therapy. Physical therapy incorporates piriformis stretching and isometric strengthening as well as modalities for pain control [16]. Foam rolling centered around the buttocks provides an excellent stretching exercise that assists in relaxation of the piriformis muscle.

Stress Fractures

Skeletally mature, active young adults are at increased risk for insufficiency fracture or stress fracture of the femoral neck, particularly young women with the "female athlete triad" consisting of an eating disorder, amenorrhea, and osteoporosis [17]. Older adults involved in endurance exercise are also at increased risk for fractures of the femur and pelvis, though they are more often affected by degenerative arthritis in the hip.

Femoral neck stress fractures can present as persistent groin pain that increases with activity. Femoral neck stress fractures can progress to unstable fractures, which are at increased risk for avascular necrosis of the femoral head. Range of motion may or not be painful, and patients may have pain with palpation of the greater trochanter. Radiographically, plain films may demonstrate cortical defects in the femoral neck. Bone scans can be very useful when ruling out stress fractures of the femoral neck, as they are up to 100% sensitive in this regard [18]. However, neither aforementioned modality is diagnostic. Magnetic resonance imaging (MRI) is more commonly used to diagnose insufficiency fractures particularly when plain films are negative. Stress fractures can be treated non-operatively with stringent non-weight-bearing protocols until the patient has clinical and radiographic evidence of healing. Some stress fractures will need to be addressed surgically with open reduction internal fixation.

Osteoarthritis and Weight Management

Osteoarthritis of the hip is a serious condition, especially in the aging athlete. The "wear and tear" of the hip joint leads to extreme pain and discomfort during activity and often prevents the aging athlete from continuing activity. Older athletes are at much greater risk of developing osteoarthritis of the hip joint, which is a major cause of disability in those of 65 years old. Several factors likely contribute to this condition, including previous acute or chronic injuries to structures around the hip, obesity, and genetic factors. End-stage degenerative joint disease (DJD) is managed surgically with total hip arthroplasty (THA). Chapter 15 of this book discusses returning to activity and sports following THA for advanced hip DJD. THA is a successful surgical treatment option; however, prior to severe degenerative changes, conservative management is recommended.

Conservative treatment options, particularly in the setting of early hip degenerative joint disease, initially include non-steroidal anti-inflammatories, physical therapy, and weight loss. Obesity is one modifiable risk factor for the development of hip osteoarthritis [19]. Furthermore, excess weight causes increased pressure within the hip joint, exacerbating symptoms of osteoarthritis [20]. Furthermore, total hip arthroplasty complications—including hardware failure rates, infection, and revision rates – significantly increase in the obese population [21]. As such, weight management can be an effective strategy to help reduce symptoms of hip degenerative joint disease and help decrease complication rates of total hip arthroplasty surgery. Corticosteroid injections can also be utilized as a secondary conservative treatment strategy. Complications associated with corticosteroid injections include elevation of blood glucose levels (particularly important in diabetic patients), local skin reactions, and potentially increased risks of infection after THA [22, 23].

References

1. Boyd KT, Peirce NS, Batt ME. Common hip injuries in sport. Sports Med. 1997;24:273–88.
2. Looney CG, Raynor B, Lowe R. Adhesive capsulitis of the hip: a review. J Am Acad Orthop Surg. 2013;21:749–55.
3. Caroit M, Djian A, Hubault A, Normandin C, De Seze S. 2 cases of retractile capsulitis of the hip [French]. Rev Rhum Mal Osteoartic. 1963;30:784–9.
4. Chard MD, Jenner JR. The frozen hip: an underdiagnosed condition. BMJ. 1988;297:596–7.

5. Lequesne M, Becker J, Bard M, Witvoet J, Postel M. Capsular constriction of the hip: arthrographic and clinical considerations. Skeletal Radiol. 1981;6:1–10.
6. Luukkainen R, Asikainen E. Frozen hip. Scand J Rheumatol. 1992;21:97.
7. Griffiths HJ, Utz R, Burke J, Bonfiglio T. Adhesive capsulitis of the hip and ankle. AJR Am J Roentgenol. 1985;144:101–5.
8. Lowe R. Adhesive capsulitis of the hip: a case report. An entity in question. Man Ther. 2013;18(6):594–7. https://doi.org/10.1016/j.smath.2012.08.006.
9. Tibor LM, Sekiya JK. Differential diagnosis of pain around the hip joint. Arthroscopy. 2008; 24:1407–21.
10. Ege Rasmussen KJ, Fano N. Trochanteric bursitis. Treatment by corticosteroid injection. Scand J Rheumatol. 1985;14:417–20.
11. Baker CL, Massie V, Hurt WG, Savory CG. Arthroscopic bursectomy for recalcitrant trochanteric bursitis. Arthroscopy. 2007;23:827–32.
12. Williams BS, Cohen SP. Greater trochanteric pain syndrome: a review of anatomy, diagnosis and treatment. Anesth Analg. 2009;108:1662–70.
13. Farr D, Selesnick H, Janecki C, Cordas D. Arthroscopic bursectomy with concomitant iliotibial band release for the treatment of recalcitrant trochanteric bursitis. Arthroscopy. 2007;23:905. e1–5.
14. Benson ER, Schutzer SF. Posttraumatic piriformis syndrome: diagnosis and results of operative treatment. J Bone Joint Surg Am. 1999;81:941–9.
15. Jankovic D, Peng P, van Zundert A. Brief review: piriformis syndrome: etiology, diagnosis and management. Can J Anaesth. 2013;60:1003–12.
16. Miller TA, White KP, Ross DC. The diagnosis and management of piriformis syndrome: myths and facts. Can J Neurol Sci. 2013;39:577–83.
17. Hilibrand MJ, Hammoud S, Bishop M, Woods D, Frederick RW, Dodson CC. Common injuries and ailments of the female athlete: pathophysiology, treatment and prevention. Phys Sportsmed. 2015;43(4):403–11.
18. Prather JL, Nusynowitz ML, Snowdy HA, Hughes AD, McCartney WH, Bagg RJ. Scintigraphic findings in stress fractures. J Bone Joint Surg Am. 1997;59:869–74.
19. Reyes C, Leyland KM, Peat G, Cooper C, Arden NK, Prieto-Alhambra D. Association between overweight and obesity and risk of clinically diagnosed knee, hip, and hand osteoarthritis: a population-based cohort study. Arthritis Rheumatol. 2016;68(8):1869–75.
20. Springer BD, Carter JT, McLawhorn AS, Scharf K, Roslin M, Kallies KJ, Morton JM, Kothari SN. Obesity and the role of bariatric surgery in the surgical management of osteoarthritis of the hipand knee: a review of the literature. Surg Obes Relat Dis. 2016;(16):30697–9. pii: S1550-7289. [Epub ahead of print].
21. George J, Klika AK, Navale SM, Newman JM, Barsoum WK, Higuera CA. Obesity epidemic: is its impact on total joint arthroplasty underestimated? An analysis of national trends. Clin Orthop Relat Res. 2017. https://doi.org/10.1007/s11999-016-5222-4. [Epub ahead of print].
22. Charalambous CP, Prodromidis AD, Kwaees TA. Do intra-articular steroid injections increase infection rates in subsequent arthroplasty? A systemic review and meta-analysis of comparative studies. J Arthroplasty. 2014;29:2175–80.
23. Ravi B, Escott BG, Wasserstein D, Croxford R, Holland S, Paterson JM, Kreder HJ, Hawker GA. Intraarticular hip injection and early revision surgery following total hip arthroplasty: a retrospective cohort study. Arthritis Rheumatol. 2015;67(1):162–8.

Chapter 10
Shoulder Injuries: Conservative Management, Operative Management, and Return to Sport

Albert Lin and Jason P. Zlotnicki

Superior Labrum and Associated Long Head Biceps Tendon Injuries

Introduction

Superior labral and long head of the biceps tendon injuries are among the most common injuries sustained in athletes. Tears of the superior labrum in an anterior to posterior direction (SLAP) tears have been extensively studied and characterized and are known to be a major cause of shoulder instability, pain, and decreased function. Special consideration must be given to the "aging athlete" population as the expectations and complications associated with management of these injuries differ in comparison to a younger population. Significant controversy, in particular, exists regarding the optimal surgical treatment of these injuries in the athlete older than 40 years when non-operative treatment has failed.

The superior labrum is an augment to the stability of the glenohumeral joint. Comprised mainly of fibrocartilaginous tissue, it serves as a bumper to multidirectional movement of the humeral head and is contiguous with the long head biceps tendon, which originates at approximately the 12 o'clock position on the glenoid. This anatomic arrangement confers particular stability of the shoulder in the externally abducted position, and its biomechanical function is often the main reason cited for the prevalence of superior labral tears and associated biceps pathology in athletes whose sport requires repetitive overhead motions [1, 2]. Several types of SLAP tears have been described. By far the most common injury that has been extensively studied is the Snyder classification, Type II tear (Fig. 10.1), which will be the main focus of this section.

A. Lin, MD (✉) · J. P. Zlotnicki, MD
Department of Orthopaedic Surgery, University of Pittsburgh Medical Center (UPMC), Pittsburgh, PA, USA
e-mail: Lina2@upmc.edu; Zlotnickijp2@upmc.edu

© Springer International Publishing AG, part of Springer Nature 2018
V. J. Wright, K. K. Middleton (eds.), *Masterful Care of the Aging Athlete*,
https://doi.org/10.1007/978-3-319-16223-2_10

95

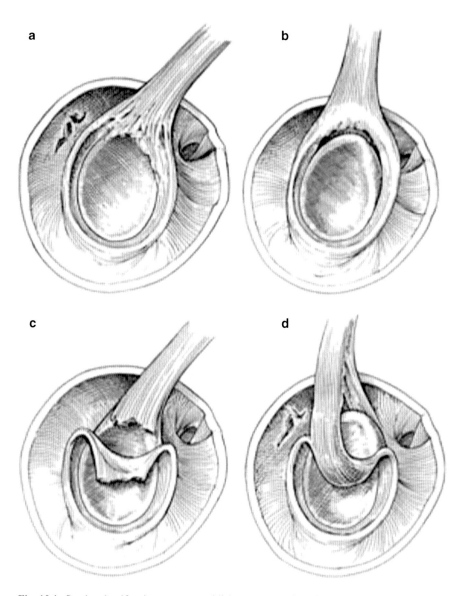

Fig. 10.1 Snyder classification system establishes a progression of degeneration and pathology. (**a**) Type I, fraying of labrum and biceps tendon with attachment preserved; (**b**) Type II, fraying with detachment of tendon anchor; (**c**) Type III, bucket handle tear of labrum with intact tendon (separation of tendon from labrum); and (**d**) Type IV, bucket handle tear with detached tendon (no separation of tendon from labrum) (Reprinted with permission from Stephen J. Snyder, Ronald P. Karzel, Wilson Del Pizzo, Richard D. Ferkel, Marc J. Friedman, SLAP lesions of the shoulder, Arthroscopy: The Journal of Arthroscopic & Related Surgery, Volume 6, Issue 4,1990, Pages 274–279)

Patient Evaluation

Different treatment modalities for SLAP tears and biceps tendinopathy exist and are aimed at the sporting activity, as well as the functional level and age of the patient. Evaluation begins with a thorough history of the shoulder disability. The patient may describe symptoms such as "clicking" or "popping" with overhead extension or during the cocking phase of throwing [2–4]. With concomitant biceps tendinopathy, the patient may also describe anterior or bicipital groove pain as well. The physical exam starts with basic shoulder mechanics, including an examination of active and passive range of motion of the glenohumeral joint and scapulothoracic joint, searching for rotational deficits or capsular tightness, such as glenohumeral internal rotational deficit (GIRD), that places excessive stress on the labrum and biceps insertion [1]. Strength is also tested at this stage. Once motion and strength have been assessed and compared to the contralateral extremity, provocative testing is performed. Many provocative tests have been described including the O'Brien's test for SLAP tears and Speed's test and bicipital groove tenderness for biceps pathology [5, 6]. It is well known, however, that while these tests are highly sensitive, they are not particularly sensitive for isolating SLAP or biceps pathology [4, 6, 7]. In addition, Keener and Brophy described how the aging athlete presentation may be confounded by concomitant shoulder pathology such as osteoarthritis of the acromioclavicular (AC) joint or the glenohumeral (GH) joint and rotator cuff pathology that can further decrease the sensitivity and specificity of the provocative physical exam maneuvers [7]. Despite numerous exam maneuvers that have been studied for isolated injuries or in combination with other pathology, no clear or convincing data exists for a highly accurate physical exam for superior labral injuries.

Imaging is often needed to confirm suspicions of a SLAP tear. The initial work-up begins with plain radiographs; standard views include a true anteroposterior, outlet, AC joint, and axillary views. These initial radiographs will not highlight labral pathology but will provide valuable information regarding other existing pathologies that may disrupt normal shoulder mechanics, such as AC joint or GH osteoarthritis. For most surgeons, MR arthrogram is the modality of choice to assess a superior labral injury. However, the timing to obtain such a study is surgeon dependent and may be based on failure of non-operative treatment, the duration of symptoms, or the level of dysfunction. Almost all studies report a sensitivity of over 90% for detecting Type II SLAP lesions (Fig. 10.2). It is important to note that a high false-positive rate has been reported with MR arthrograms [8, 9]. While an ABER position on coronal oblique can help to lower this false-positive rate [10], it cannot be overstated that only in combination with a detailed history and physical examination will an MRI arthrogram be useful in confirming a diagnosis.

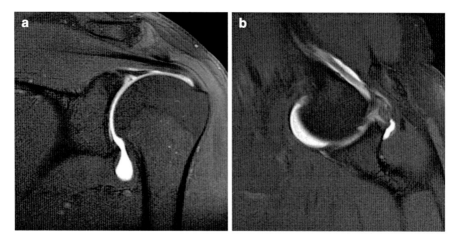

Fig. 10.2 MR arthrogram of 40-year-old male active duty in the air force, with classic symptoms of a SLAP tear. (**a**) Coronal T2 arthrogram showing extravasation of contrast fluid under the tear. (**b**) ABER view T2 arthrogram image demonstrating superior labral tear

Non-operative Management and Return to Sport

The initial step in managing superior labrum and biceps pathology is a trial of conservative treatment, specifically tailored to regaining strength, ROM, and proprioception of the rotator cuff muscles and scapula. This includes a standard rest period or break from sporting activity; physical therapy aimed at specific pathology and concomitant shoulder pathology, strength, and ROM; and nonsteroidal anti-inflammatory medications. In the younger cohort, physical therapy appears to be successful in a small number of patients with the least severe (Type I) SLAP injuries. A study was performed by Edwards et al. in which athletes with an average age of 34 ± 9 years were found to have significant functional improvement when followed for an average of 3.1 years from start of non-operative management [11]. Pain relief and functional improvement were achieved compared to pretreatment; and return to sports was successful, but athletes were not able to return to overhead activities at pre-injury level. For the aging athlete, however, there are no high-quality studies assessing the duration and types of conservative treatment and the overall effectiveness of conservative management. Further studies that examine non-operative outcomes for isolated SLAP lesions, as well as SLAP lesions with concomitant pathology, are needed to characterize this treatment paradigm. Nonetheless, a trial of conservative treatment is often recommended before operative consideration.

Operative Management and Return to Sport

Once conservative treatment has failed, the athlete is an appropriate candidate for surgical management. Multiple surgical treatments have been described including primary repair, biceps tenodesis, biceps tenotomy, and labral debridement. The selection of a particular surgery is based on features of the individual disease pathology as well as the age of the patient. High success rates for primary Type II SLAP repair have been reported in the younger population, with >90% achievement of "good to excellent" results [2, 12]. There are, however, multiple studies that suggest this trend does not carry over to the aging athlete population. A recent review by Erickson et al. found that although similar results were seen in some studies between the <40-year-old and >40-year-old cohorts, other studies observed significant higher failure rates in the older cohort for primary SLAP repair. The main complications observed were overall decreased patient satisfaction, increased postoperative stiffness, and increased reoperation rates [13]. Although observed success rates varied between studies in the aforementioned review, a pervasive theme observed was that aging, overhead athletes do not report consistent satisfaction and function after arthroscopic repair [13–16].

Over the past 15 years, a new paradigm of treatment has emerged in which biceps tenodesis and tenotomy are effective (and sometimes superior) alternatives to operative repair of Type II SLAP lesions, particularly for the aging athlete. Studies comparing SLAP repair to biceps tenodesis in the 40 years plus cohort demonstrated significantly improved functional scores, increased satisfaction, and higher rates of return to previous level of sports participation with tenodesis [14, 17]. Similarly, both biceps tenotomy and tenodesis were reported to be reliable alternatives to SLAP repair, with both procedures acceptable for revision SLAP repair. Moreover, tenotomy/tenodesis may be more effective in the aging athlete when labral pathology is present with concomitant rotator cuff injury [18–21]. A recent study evaluated the management of failed SLAP lesions, comparing nonsurgical and surgical options. Considering that aging athletes are likely to have had previous procedures to address shoulder pathology and that SLAP repair failures often leave patients with limited options, the study found that a revision to a biceps tenodesis was a valuable salvage with successful outcomes in this particular setting [22]. In a similar light, Franceschi et al. reported on patients undergoing rotator cuff repairs with concomitant SLAP tears, comparing SLAP repair and biceps tenotomy. Both cohorts demonstrated improvement with no significant advantage of a SLAP repair, leading to the overall conclusion that a SLAP repair was not particularly warranted given the risks of SLAP repair failure and subsequent complications [23].

Despite the evidence for caution with primary SLAP repair in the aging athlete, the impact on clinical practice for both young and aging athletes alike is unclear. Zhang et al. performed a descriptive epidemiologic study of surgeons that showed orthopedic surgeons are performing more SLAP repairs each year, with the highest incidence of repair in the 20–29- and 40–49-year age groups [24]. However, more recently, Patterson et al. showed with a query of the American Boards of Orthopaedic Surgery (ABOS) part II database study that the frequency of SLAP repair is decreasing, with an increase in biceps tenodesis and tenotomy, documenting that an increased patient age correlates with the likelihood of treatment with tenodesis/tenotomy versus primary SLAP repair [25].The overall trend in the literature appears to support tenodesis or tenotomy as a more favorable procedure regarding improved patient outcomes and return to sport in the aging athlete. However, at this time, there is still no clear consensus.

Conclusion

In the aging athlete, there is a wide range of superior labral and biceps tendon pathologies that is unique to each athlete, their level of pre-pathology function, and their chosen sport. It is common for concomitant pathology to exist in the presence of SLAP lesions, making diagnosis and treatment more difficult. The evaluation of any aging athlete includes a thorough history, a targeted and organized physical exam, and selection of the proper imaging modality. A combination of history, exam, and imaging is more successful in diagnosis and directing the appropriate treatment than any in isolation. A trial of non-operative treatment is indicated for most SLAP tears, with an understanding that a return to sport from a more severe injury and return to overhead activities may be less successful. Operative management can be successful for SLAP tears and biceps pathology, although tenodesis or tenotomy of the biceps tendon appears to offer improved outcomes with less stiffness and post-op complications than primary repair in the aging athlete. Despite the growing body of research, there is a need for new outcomes focused research on the non-operative and operative management of the aging athlete as no clear consensus currently exists.

Shoulder Dislocation and Concomitant Injury in the Aging Athlete

Introduction

In older patients, shoulder dislocations often present with an array of complex injury patterns when compared to the same injury in the younger population. Owing to its wide range of motion, the shoulder is the most commonly dislocated large joint in the body, with reported incidence as high as 23.9 per 100,000 persons/year [26, 27]. Shoulder dislocations occur in a bimodal distribution with the highest prevalence found between the ages of 10–20 and 50–60 years old [28, 29]. However, there is significantly more research on the younger population due to the risk of recurrent dislocation, with recurrence rates reported from 92 to 96% in young athletes <30 years old [30–32]. This difference in rate of recurrence is a result of joint differences between young and older populations and the overall mechanism of dislocation.

In general, younger athletes experience an "anterior structure-related mechanism" of injury in which the weaker anterior static restraints fail as opposed to healthy rotator cuff tissue; this often results in a labral tear following a first-time traumatic dislocation, such as a classic Bankart lesion [33]. Conversely, the aging athlete has weaker dynamic constraints (rotator cuff) due to aging and chronic degeneration and will therefore frequently present with an accompanying rotator cuff tear usually with no labral tear or Bankart lesion present [34]. Values are variable in the literature, but reported rates of a rotator cuff tear with anterior dislocation in the >40-year-old patient population range from 30 to 70%, with smaller studies even reporting 100% tear rates with dislocation [35–40]. Studies have shown that older patients have higher rates of concomitant fractures of the humerus and neurovascular injuries as well [41]. The risk of recurrent dislocation events is less frequent in the older population, but pain and loss of function can persist in the event of damage to neighboring anatomy. In the following sections, shoulder dislocations in the aging athlete will be further examined, with discussion regarding the initial work-up, management paradigms, and the best evidence for functional restoration and return to sport. Particular attention will be paid to concomitant rotator cuff injuries.

Patient Evaluation

Initial evaluation of the athlete with a present or past dislocation begins with a detailed history regarding the traumatic event, assessing for any noticeable neurovascular deficits, and simple observation. Given that approximately 90–100% of traumatic shoulder dislocations are anterior [30], the patient will likely present with the arm held fixed, internally rotated, and abducted if acutely dislocated. Since the shoulder may be adequately reduced on presentation, a dislocation diagnosis can be overlooked in the absence of obvious deformity or deficit and lead to an inaccurate work-up and treatment. In the acute setting of a dislocation, prior to any manipulation or physical examination, radiographic examination is warranted. Standard shoulder films, including an AP view and, in particular, an axillary view, are obtained to assess for a reduced humeral head and acute fracture of the glenoid or greater tuberosity. In the event of a reduced joint without acute fracture, close attention should be paid to survey for evidence of past dislocation such as erosions or fracture, which will influence further work-up and management. CT scan and MRI are not routinely indicated in the acute presentation in an emergency department but will detect subtle fractures and characterize the integrity of the neighboring soft tissues.

Physical examination of the patient after reduction should assess joint stability, status of neurovascular structures, and active and passive ROM, with a thorough examination of the rotator cuff [42]. As discussed above, the pathophysiology of dislocation in the aging athlete increases the likelihood of an accompanying injury. Robinson et al. reported in 2012 that of 3633 traumatic dislocations, 40% of patients had an associated structural injury about the GH joint, 33% sustained a RC tear or greater tuberosity fracture, and 13% experienced neurological injury, most commonly the axillary nerve [39]. An earlier study by Toolanen showed similar high rates of concomitant injury, specifically in patients with persistent pain and symptoms at follow-up [43]. The likelihood of recurrent instability or dislocations in patients over 40 years old is much less common compared to their <20-year-old cohorts [28], though a grossly unstable shoulder may be an indication for an MRI as a massive RC tear may be present. Close attention should be paid to complaints of instability and pain weeks to months after a trauma. A systematic review by Gomberawalla et al. showed that persistent pain and dysfunction after a shoulder dislocation often accompanied rotator cuff tears, especially in contact or overhead athletes, patients older than 40 years, or those with nerve injury [43, 44]. Given the much higher rates of concomitant injuries in older athletes, particularly of the rotator cuff, advanced imaging with a prompt MRI is usually indicated as these injuries may be relatively time sensitive in terms of progression and further treatment. Prompt radiographs, assessment of stability, strength and RC function, and neurovascular evaluation are mandatory in the aging athlete status post shoulder dislocation.

Non-operative Management

Acute management of the shoulder dislocation in the aging athlete is no different than a younger athlete; prompt recognition and closed reduction of the dislocation is necessary. Persistent dislocation can compromise the blood supply to the humeral head, cause nerve damage, and necessitate an open approach for reduction. Most reductions can be performed under sedation or an intra-articular block, which helps to reduce muscular spasm allowing for a less traumatic reduction. If the dislocation is chronic (days to weeks), closed reduction may be extremely challenging and an open reduction may be indicated. A study by Stayner in 2000 evaluating outcomes of closed reductions for acute shoulder dislocations in emergency departments found that 88% of patients achieved uneventful closed reduction in the ED, 5% needed general anesthesia for closed reduction, and only 3% required open reduction [45].

In the subacute clinical setting, initial treatment is non-operative and focuses on restoring the musculature and dynamic stabilizers of the shoulder. This is done while allowing for healing of injured static structures and assuming no concomitant fractures or associated traumatic rotator cuff tear. However, it may be difficult to ascertain whether an accompanying rotator cuff lesion caused instability or a dislocation event leads to acute rupture [46]. This decision must be based on presenting symptoms and physical exam, as a patient with minimal pain and lack of reproducible instability despite a rotator cuff injury may be considered for non-operative management [47]. Early range of motion exercises and physical therapy are usually recommended to avoid posttraumatic stiffness and loss of motion while retaining glenohumeral stability [48]. Pendulum exercises and progressive passive/active motion can be effective in achieving motion, return of function, and relief of pain in patients without a concomitant rotator cuff tear.

The aging athlete cohort is less likely to need operative management for labral pathology, as rotator cuff pathology is much more common. Despite accompanying pathology, patients over 50 have a significantly lower chance of developing recurrent instability compared to their younger cohorts [28], which allows safe initiation of therapy in the absence of gross instability or pseudoparalysis. Development of these latter symptoms was previously attributed either to nerve palsy or described as the "terrible shoulder triad" [49] but is now more frequently realized as concomitant rotator cuff injury in review of the literature [44]. Presently, there are no clear studies demonstrating overall functional recovery or return to sport in the aging athlete population following non-operative management of a dislocation. Therefore, there is no consensus regarding the duration and frequency of physical therapy needed or the amount of time recommended before increasing activity and returning to sport. Patients are generally allowed to progress with activity in the absence of pain or loss of motion and strength and can return to sport when those milestones are met.

Operative Management

Conversely, patients who fail physical therapy in terms of pain or recurrent instability and who have persistent rotator cuff weakness will often require additional MRI evaluation and may need operative repair. Because of the high prevalence of traumatic rotator cuff tears in patients >40 years old, many orthopedic surgeons often recommend prompt assessment with an MRI prior to initiating conservative treatment (Fig. 10.3). It is generally accepted that early diagnosis and repair of traumatic rotator cuff tears lead to optimal outcomes and the best return of function [44, 50]. Further evidence suggests that early surgical repair results in improved pain relief and patient satisfaction compared to non-operative management, and repair of accompanying capsular lesions helps restore shoulder stability [51, 52]. However, a

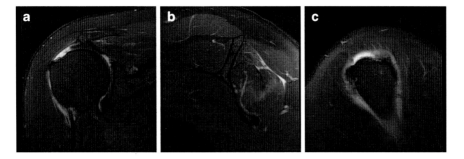

Fig. 10.3 MRI of 45-year-old male postreduction after acute dislocation while playing basketball. (**a**) Coronal T2 image showing classic rotator cuff rupture with small amount of preserved insertional cuff tissue, (**b**) T2 sagittal image showing enhancement of the infraspinatus muscle belly consistent with acute inflammation and rupture, (**c**) T2 sagittal image showing the extent of the tear in the anterior-to-posterior direction

recent study by Maier in 2009 found that while operative repair of rotator cuff lesions reduced the rate of recurrent instability in both older (age > 40 years old) and younger patients, clinical functional outcomes were significantly worse in the older cohort [53]. Persistent dysfunction in the older individual is rarely related to recurrent instability but is rather related to progressive sequelae following an untreated traumatically ruptured rotator cuff. However, while the current literature suggests improved stability and function after surgical repair of the rotator cuff, there is no consensus for operative management, specific patient indications, or functional return to play after operative repair of the rotator cuff after dislocations. In a study performed by Shin et al. in 2012 which evaluated non-operative rehab patients (no rotator cuff tear) versus operative patients (concomitant cuff tear), patients who were treated non-operatively showed significantly better recovery of shoulder function than patients who were treated operatively [54]. While this data does not evaluate operative versus non-operative management in the setting of a concomitant cuff tear, it does provide useful prognostic information for patients with a rotator cuff tear associated with their dislocation. At this time, there is limited data regarding return to sport following operative management for shoulder dislocations in the aging athlete.

Conclusions

In the event of a traumatic dislocation of the shoulder in the aging athlete, prompt reduction is a priority to avoid neurovascular injury or associated bony injury. Radiographic studies should be obtained prior to and after all reductions in the acute setting. In the subacute setting, a focused history and physical examination is a priority as shoulder dislocations can be missed if the patient presents with a reduced shoulder. In cases of acute traumatic dislocation, there is a high prevalence of concomitant rotator cuff tear, fractures, and nerve disruption in the aging athlete. Initial treatment after reduction should focus on regaining function of dynamic stabilizers of the shoulder and range of motion. In cases of persistent shoulder pain with weakness or a traumatic rotator cuff tear, operative repair of the rotator cuff is often indicated. However, there is a lack of high-quality evidence documenting functional outcomes and return to sport for non-operative versus operative management in this particular setting. There is a need for further, prospective research regarding functional outcomes after management of traumatic dislocations, with or without rotator cuff injury, in aging athletes, regarding return to pre-injury level of function.

Rotator Cuff and Subacromial Impingement

Introduction

Impingement and rotator cuff disease are common causes of shoulder pain in the aging athlete. Persistent repetitive compression of the rotator cuff due to primary mechanical subacromial impingement may lead to fraying and eventual tearing of the rotator cuff if left untreated. Intrinsic degeneration of the rotator cuff is also known to occur as a result of the normal aging process with higher rates of incidental tears found in progressively older individuals [55]. While impingement syndrome and degenerative rotator cuff tears have been theorized to develop as a result of unfavorable shoulder mechanics and chronic degeneration, rotator cuff injuries in the aging athlete can also present with acute trauma, with either sudden or acute on chronic onset. Special consideration must be given to the "aging athlete" in both instances, as early diagnosis and management is essential to optimize outcomes. In older individuals, management is often complicated by concomitant shoulder pathology, making diagnosis more difficult and treatment goals less clear. Most importantly, limited evidence is present regarding non-operative and operative treatment paradigms of symptomatic and asymptomatic injuries in the aging athlete, and little is known regarding functional outcomes and return to sport. This section will outline the work-up of a patient with suspected subacromial impingement or rotator cuff pathology and the current evidence for indications and functional outcomes of operative and non-operative treatment.

Patient Evaluation

Evaluation starts with a thorough history of the timeframe and any recent traumatic insult. The age of the patient, sporting activity, and his/her current level of function may also influence decision-making and treatment. Often the patient will present with complaints of lateral aching pain but deny any specific event or inciting cause for the shoulder pain. Patients are often unable to "isolate" or "pinpoint" a specific area of pain but, rather, describe a region of pain near the lateral upper third of the arm near the deltoid insertion [56]. Specific complaints may include nocturnal pain and significant difficulty and aggravation of symptoms with overhead activities, which are common complaints for both subacromial impingement and rotator cuff pathology alike. These non-specific but frequent symptoms may alert the surgeon to possible rotator cuff pathology and aid in the physical exam assessment to clarify the clinical picture. Athletes who engage in repetitive overhead sports in particular such as swimming and racquet sports may be more susceptible to pathology. However, not all rotator cuff injuries are chronic, as acute rupture can also occur. This distinction is difficult, because the presence of new-onset symptoms, suggestive of an acute process in the aging athlete, does not rule out the presence of a chronic tear that has propagated and now become symptomatic. Therefore, it is important to note the emergence of acute, new-onset symptoms as a clinically significant entity that may require more acute, less conservative management.

The physical exam starts with evaluation of basic shoulder mechanics, including active and passive range of motion, and assessment of rotator cuff strength. The shoulder must be exposed, along with the contralateral limb, to evaluate for any muscular atrophy indicative of chronicity. Motion may be limited actively, but a patient with impingement or rotator cuff injury should achieve relatively full (although sometimes painful) passive motion. The classic "painful flexion arc" is commonly observed, where symptoms are present with the arm in forward flexion with worsening pain as the arm reaches parallel to ground level and remains as it is moved overhead. Stiffness may be observed with partial-thickness rotator cuff tears, which leads to pain, loss of motion, and relative joint contracture [57]. If examination yields severe loss of both active and passive motion, additional shoulder pathology must be considered, including osteoarthritis of the glenohumeral joint or adhesive capsulitis. Strength testing is paramount, as each of the rotator cuff muscles can be individually isolated and classified by the commonly used Oxford scale (0–5/5 scale) or with dynamometer. Once strength has been characterized, rotator cuff "lag signs" are assessed and may better characterize a tear as partial or full thickness [58, 59]. A full description of all lag signs is beyond the scope of this section; however, these lag signs are generally present with more severe pathology including large, full-thickness rotator cuff tears or chronic full-thickness tears [59].

Provocative maneuvers are next assessed. The Neer and Hawkins impingement maneuvers are often performed and are sensitive, but not specific for impingement and rotator cuff pathology. These tests however are a good starting point for evaluating irritation of the rotator cuff (identifying all partial- and full-thickness tears) and tend to be positive for subacromial impingement as well [60]. Further evaluation may be gathered from the "impingement test" in which provocative testing is repeated after a subacromial injection of anesthetic. Though less commonly done in practice, relief of pain after injection confirms a subacromial lesion, and persistent weakness regardless of pain suggests a full-thickness tendon injury. Individual tests, such as the Jobe ("empty can") test, have been studied for sensitivity and specificity with no clear demonstration of a single, conclusive test. A recent systematic review by Hermans et al. in *Journal of the American Medical Association* (*JAMA*) reported that a positive painful arc test and positive external rotation resistance test were most accurate for detecting disease of the rotator cuff, while positive lag signs (either external or internal lag) were most accurate for the diagnosis of a full-thickness rotator cuff tear [61].

Imaging begins with a plain radiographic impingement series; axillary view, scapular outlet, and true AP. Chronic tears of the rotator cuff may show greater tuberosity changes, including cysts that may mirror subacromial undersurface bone spurring. Acromion morphology can be further classified, based on shape, as a Type I (flat), Type II (curved), and Type III (hooked) using a classification first described by Bigliani [62]. Subacromial findings may be prominent, yet the relevance of these findings remains controversial. A recent study by Chalal et al. suggested no difference in outcomes with isolated bursal resection versus modification of the acromial anatomy [63]. For most, the imaging modality of choice for diagnosis of a rotator cuff tear is an magnetic resonance imaging (MRI) or an magnetic resonance arthrography (MRA). Recent review articles demonstrate a sensitivity/specificity of 98 and 79% for the detection of any rotator cuff tear with MRI, while MRA demonstrates a sensitivity/specificity of 94 and 92% for the detection of full-thickness lesions [64]. Specific characteristics of a tear may also be accurately assessed with an MRI including tear size, degree of tendon retraction, the presence of fat infiltration of the involved muscle, and concomitant pathology. Ultrasound is emerging as a potential alternative to MRI with certain studies suggesting sensitivity and specificity of preoperative ultrasound to be >90%, with no significant difference from MRI in detecting the presence of a tear [64, 65]. However, these results are variable and user dependent.

Partial tears may be articular sided or bursal sided, with articular-sided tears being approximately 3–4 times more prevalent. From prior studies, both clinical and cadaveric, partial-thickness tears are more common than full-thickness tears, and overhead athletes or laborers tend to develop articular-sided, partial-thickness tears. Tears that involve more than 50% of the insertional footprint are considered "high grade" and may eventually require surgical fixation (Fig. 10.4). The specific age of the aging athlete is an important consideration, as full-thickness tears are more common after the fifth and sixth decades of life [57]. In summary, the age of the patient, chronicity of pathology, and presence of a partial- versus full-thickness tear are key components of the work-up that help inform non-operative and operative treatment options.

Non-operative Management and Return to Sport

For impingement syndrome or a degenerative rotator cuff tear, particularly in older individuals, initial treatment generally begins with a course of non-operative management including rest, activity modification, and nonsteroidal anti-inflammatory drugs [66]. Physical therapy is often initiated. A subacromial corticosteroid injection for

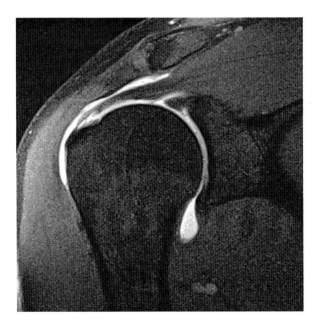

Fig. 10.4 A 36-year-old male who sustained acute injury to right shoulder while snowboarding. MRI arthrogram, T2 coronal, demonstrates a high-grade, near full-thickness, partial articular-sided supraspinatus tear involving greater than 50% of overall insertional footprint

impingement syndrome may also be beneficial. Both physical therapy and steroid treatments have been shown to achieve significant improvement in impingement syndrome patients, with approximately 50% improvement observed and maintained through 1 year without a significant difference observed between therapy and injection [67].

There continues to be limited outcomes data on non-operative management of partial- and full-thickness tears. However, most patients will experience improvement of pain and function within 6 months [66]. One of the most documented complications of non-operative therapy is tear progression, which has been observed in the natural history of both symptomatic and asymptomatic lesions [68, 69]. This is significant as increased tear size, increased time to management, and poorer muscle quality are associated with worse surgical outcomes irrespective of patient age and functional status [70, 71]. With non-operative management of massive full-thickness tears, Zingg et al. showed that patients can maintain satisfactory shoulder function for at least 4 years. However, there is a significant risk of a reparable tear progressing to an irreparable tear within this same time period [72]. A recent study by Moosmayer et al. comparing non-operative and operative management demonstrated that primary operative repair of small- and medium-sized rotator cuff tears yielded better functional outcomes than rehabilitation, but these effects were small enough to question the clinical significance. Complicating matters further, this study also demonstrated that in a small subset of patients, increasing tear size was observed in the non-operative group, which was associated with poor functional outcomes over the 5 years of the study [73].

A more recent study attempted to clarify which patients are better suited for non-operative management with less risk of tear progression. Fucentese et al. demonstrated that while larger tears were known to progress and can do so in a short amount of time, single tendon tears—hence, smaller-sized lesions—showed significantly decreased rates of progression with no increase in tear size. They propose that smaller full-thickness tears may be better managed with non-operative therapy with less risk of tear progression [74]. Nonetheless, there remains a lack of data evaluating return to sport following non-operative management of rotator cuff tears.

Operative Management and Return to Sport

Operative management is generally recommended whenever conservative therapies are ineffective. Despite numerous articles that endorse pain relief and improved function with surgical treatment [75–79], recent controversial studies have implied that surgical treatment with arthroscopic subacromial decompression may not be more effective than active exercises and non-operative management in reducing pain intensity in patients with subacromial impingement syndrome [80, 81]. In regard to the aging population, Biberthaler et al. recently demonstrated significant improvement in patients older than 57 years compared to physical therapy [76]. In a recent study, Klintberg et al. showed that a high degree of satisfaction, including alleviation of pain and preservation of motion, was seen up to 8–11 years after arthroscopic decompression [79]. Nevertheless, operative treatment for isolated subacromial impingement remains a controversial topic. Higher-level studies are needed regarding specific recommendations and return to sport paradigms following subacromial decompression.

Studies on the natural history of rotator cuff tears showed that a large proportion of the population can have asymptomatic lesions [55, 68, 69] and that there is no current evidence that a prophylactic repair prevents long-term clinical deterioration [82]. However, certain tears such as anterior supraspinatus tears are more likely to progress over time and may warrant surgical consideration. The onset or progression of pain is often correlated with tear propagation, and these patients generally require close evaluation with considerations of early repair [83]. Regardless, ideal candidates for operative intervention typically fit into one of two categories: (1) a *symptomatic, painful* degenerative rotator cuff tear that has undergone proper work-up and a trial of non-operative treatment and (2) an acute, traumatic rotator cuff rupture.

When considering operative repair in the aging athlete, increasing age is a negative predictor for healing after repair with higher rates of recurrent tear occurring in the masters athlete population [84]. Furthermore, healing is not always correlated with a successful clinical outcome as a recent study demonstrated successful outcomes at 10 years following known structurally failed repairs [85]. In general, most studies demonstrate successful outcomes with clinical improvement in pain relief and functional outcome for the repair of both partial- and full-thickness rotator cuff lesions. Recently, Shin et al. showed that articular-sided partial-thickness tears exceeding 50% of tendon thickness showed statistically significant functional improvement and pain relief regardless of repair technique [86]. However, for full-thickness tears, the size of the tear may be more predictive of outcome than demographics or even the repair method used. Ide et al. demonstrated that arthroscopic and open repair of full-thickness, small-sized, and medium-sized tears was equivalent. There was, however, a statistically significant decrease in postoperative function in the large-massive tear group, compared to the small-medium group, with no significant difference between the arthroscopic and open technique groups [87].

Though an in-depth discussion of the various operative repair techniques is beyond the scope of this chapter, it is important to understand the functional and biomechanical analysis associated with both open and arthroscopic repair. From a functional standpoint, recent literature showed that the clinical results are similar, with no significant differences found in functional outcome or complication rate [88]. However, re-tear rates for large tears (greater than 3 cm) were shown to be more common with arthroscopic surgery compared to open procedures [89]. Open repair and mini-open repair techniques with transosseous fixation are considered the gold standard secondary to limited tendon to tuberosity motion and better replication of the supraspinatus tendon footprint [90, 91]. Multiple arthroscopic fixation methods exist including single- versus double-row fixation, traditional double-row versus "transosseous equivalent," and knotless double-row techniques. Currently, double-row fixation has been shown to be mechanically favorable more so than single-row fixation in cadaveric studies. However, clinically, no significant difference in functional outcomes has been observed with the exception that double-row repairs may be more successful in the management of large/massive (greater than 3 cm) tears with lower re-tear rates [92–95]. A more recent study performed by McCormick et al. demonstrated statistically significant improvement in both subjective and objective shoulder outcomes, with no significant difference in functional testing, range-of-motion, strength, or re-tear rates when comparing single-row, double-row, or an arthroscopic transosseous equivalent repair [96]. When comparing open or mini-open techniques to arthroscopic repair, there was no significant difference in clinical outcome based on the most recent meta-analysis of the literature [97].

Regardless of the specific operative technique, postoperative rehabilitation is important in regaining motion and function. However, there is no clear consensus as to whether early or late motion is optimal for regaining function. A recent meta-analysis by Chang et al. reported that early range-of-motion exercise accelerated recovery from stiffness but was likely to increase the rate of improper healing with large-sized tears when compared to delayed passive range-of-motion rehabilitation. Contrarily, previous studies suggested no negative effect nor decreased rates of healing with early motion [98]. Such contradictory findings highlight that the decision for early versus late motion must be made on an individual patient basis understanding the risk factors for recurrent tears [99]. Other analyses showed no clinically significant difference in early versus late motion [100].

Regarding acute ruptures of the rotator cuff, optimal outcomes were observed with early intervention. Bassett and Cofield reported superior outcomes regarding maximum shoulder function and strength with early surgical repair within 3 weeks of an acute injury [101]. More recent work by Lähteenmäki et al. demonstrated an increase in shoulder abduction and improvements in strength compared to preoperative values with maintenance of overall high level of patient function and satisfaction [102]. Lastly, a large review of the literature regarding time to surgical intervention proposes better functional outcomes with earlier operative intervention with acute RC tears [103].

The overall consensus for the aging athlete is that surgical intervention remains the mainstay for patients with continued symptoms and loss of function despite non-operative therapies. As with non-operative treatment, there is minimal evidence regarding return to sport following repair in the aging athlete. As such, recommendations for return to sport are made case by case based on individual patient characteristics and level of activity.

Conclusions

The aging athlete poses specific, unique challenges when presenting with symptoms of impingement and rotator cuff pathology. Advanced age, baseline shoulder mechanics, and the presence of early degenerative changes all make diagnosis and optimal treatment more difficult. Diagnosis of shoulder impingement and rotator cuff disease requires a thorough history and physical examination, along with provocative exam techniques and advanced imaging modalities. Management of this patient population generally begins with non-operative rehabilitation; however non-operative treatment can risk worsening disease with progression of tear size and, in some, development of an irreparable situation with prolonged loss of function. Therefore, surgical intervention at an early time point for some aging athletes, particularly for acute injuries, may be necessary for healing and restoration of function. There are limited studies that discuss the aging athlete and return to sport for both non-operative and operative management. Management should be aimed at the alleviation of pain and restoration of function and must be tailored on an individual basis to the athlete in question. For paradigms regarding return, more research is needed to clarify the natural history of operative and non-operative treatments in the aging athlete population.

Acromioclavicular Dislocation and Instability

Introduction

The acromioclavicular (AC) joint is comprised of the lateral edge of the clavicle and medial edge of the acromion. AC joint injuries are common injuries in the athletic population, representing 40–50% of athletic shoulder injuries [104]. Common mechanisms include a direct blow or fall onto the affected shoulder. The AC joint itself is comprised of both dynamic and static stabilizers. The static stabilizers consist of the joint capsule, the overlying AC ligaments, and a pair of coracoclavicular (CC) ligaments (conoid and trapezoid) (Fig. 10.5). The AC

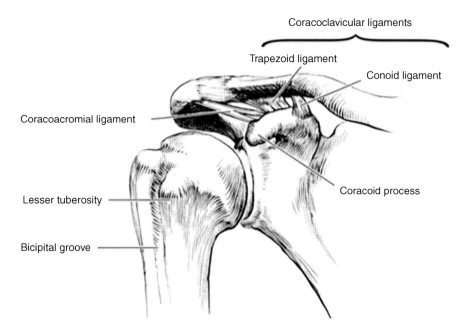

Fig. 10.5 The acromioclavicular joint, including the coracoacromial and coracoclavicular ligament complex (trapezoid and conoid) (From Simovitch R, Sanders B, Ozbaydar M, Lavery K, Warner JJ. Acromioclavicular joint injuries: diagnosis and management. J Am Acad Orthop Surg. 2009 Apr;17(4):207–19)

joint capsule confers anteroposterior stability, while the CC ligaments provide strong vertical stability of the clavicle. Injury to the CC ligaments, in particular, is important for classification. Objective grading is performed with the Rockwood classification and is scaled from Grade I through Grade VI (Fig. 10.6). Type I and II injuries commonly respond well to non-operative therapy, while Types IV–VI require surgical reconstruction. Type III injuries, however, are controversial regarding non-operative versus operative management. Despite the fact that AC injuries account for 9% of all shoulder girdle injuries, there remains a lack of evidence regarding current treatments for athletes with AC joint dislocations, with even less evidence evaluating functional recovery and return to sport in the aging athlete population. In the following section, the evaluation of AC joint dislocation injuries will be discussed, and evidence-based literature for the management, functional recovery, and rates of return to sport will be presented.

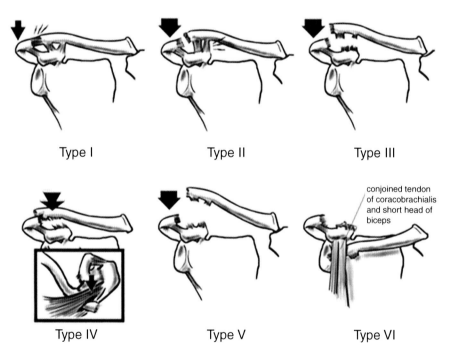

Fig. 10.6 Rockwood's classification of acromioclavicular separations Types I to VI is shown. A Type I injury is a mild sprain of the AC ligament; Type II is a ruptured AC ligament and sprained CC ligaments; Type III is a superior dislocation of the AC joint with ruptured AC ligament, CC ligament, and joint capsule; Type IV is a posterior dislocation of the AC joint with ruptured AC ligament, CC ligament, and joint capsule; Type V is a gross superior dislocation of the AC joint with ruptured AC ligament, CC ligament, and joint capsule; and Type VI is an inferior dislocation of the AC joint with rupture of the AC ligament, CC ligament, and joint capsule (Reprinted with permission from Lasanianos NG, Panteli M. Acromioclavicular (AC) joint dislocation. In: Lasanianos NG, Kanakaris NK, Giannoudis PV, eds. Trauma and Orthopaedic Classifications. London, UK: Springer-Verlag London; 2015:3–6)

Patient Evaluation

Patient examination begins with a thorough history and physical examination. Information regarding the type of injury and the mechanism are significant for assessing the level of energy. It is also important to know the daily activities of the patient. Manual laborers, as well as all aging athletes, are known to place high amounts of stress and demand on their AC joints which have historically lead to some physicians considering surgical intervention more frequently in these groups [105]. Examination of the AC joint should be performed with the contralateral shoulder exposed for comparison. Often, the deformity is clearly apparent with prominent AC joint asymmetry [106]. Severe gross deformity with tenting of overlying structures is a key sign for the acute presentation of Types IV and V dislocation. Close attention should be paid to an impending open fracture. Pain is usually present both in the acute and chronic settings. Palpation of the joint and provocative maneuvers may elicit tenderness. Athletes with chronic AC joint instability can present with stiffness of their affected shoulder [106], but most patients will show an unaffected ROM. However, if stiffness is present, further evaluation is warranted to rule out an additional underlying intracapsular pathology. A patient with chronic AC joint instability may complain of an overall ache or pain located in the medial scapula as a result of improper scapulothoracic mechanics. Both passive and active ROM will cause pain at the AC joint, which is often accentuated by provocative tests that include shoulder abduction, cross-body adduction, and the O'Brien active compression test [106, 107]. Once pain has been well localized and differentiated from non-AC joint locations, stability of the AC joint is assessed. In the acute phase, this can be very difficult due to pain and is often better assessed after 1–2 weeks of sling management and rest. Both horizontal and vertical stability must be assessed and can be a key determinate to distinguish whether an injury is severe enough to warrant surgical consideration. A Type III injury can often be reduced, which differentiates this level of injury from Type IV, V, and VI injuries [107].

Radiographic evaluation of the AC joint is achieved with plain radiographs. Anteroposterior and axial views of the shoulder comprise standard evaluation. The Zanca view, performed by tilting the XR beam approximately 10–15° in the cephalad direction, is crucial and provides the most accurate assessment of pathology secondary to the resulting clear view of the AC joint. Weighted and non-weighted views may be obtained. Joint space widening and increased coracoclavicular distance are indicative of pathology and must be compared to the contralateral side to obtain an accurate assessment (Fig. 10.7). Osteolysis of the distal clavicle or degenerative changes of the AC joint may be observed. An axial view is crucial to assess for any posterior displacement of the clavicle (Fig. 10.8). Final diagnosis and grade of the AC separation are determined following radiographic evaluation in conjunction with the history and physical exam.

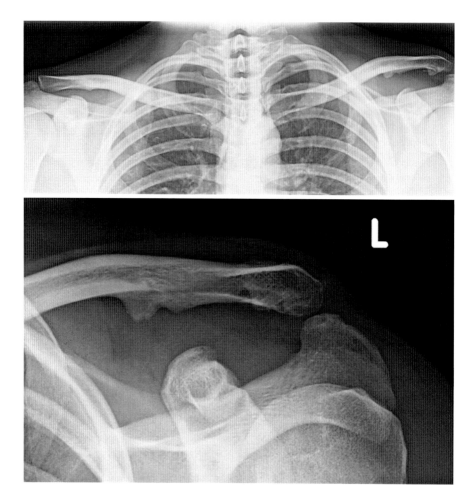

Fig. 10.7 A 29-year-old male with chronic, Type III acromioclavicular joint dislocation. Top: bilateral comparison view demonstrates increased coracoclavicular distance on affected side (left). Bottom: Zanca view of the affected AC joint, demonstrating chronic heterotopic changes at the prior coracoclavicular ligament insertion sites on the clavicle

Non-operative Management and Return to Sport

In review of the literature, it is widely accepted that Type I and II injuries are managed non-operatively and Types IV–VI should be treated operatively, preferably less than 2 to 3 weeks after an injury [108]. As stated above, the optimal treatment of Type III injuries is controversial and has undergone a paradigm shift in the past several decades. In the 1970s, surgical treatment of Type III AC joint dislocations was commonplace, but by the early 1990s, nonsurgical management was preferred by 72.2% of surgeons surveyed [109]. The currently accepted non-operative treatment protocol consists of a brief period of immobilization in a sling to limit stress

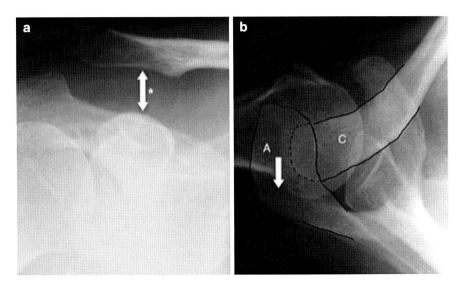

Fig. 10.8 X-ray views of a Type IV AC joint dislocation. (**a**) Zanca view demonstrated widening of the joint space and increased coracoclavicular distance. (**b**) Axillary view demonstrates posterior translation of the clavicle (C) to the acromion (A), indicative of button holing through the deltotrapezial fascia (From Simovitch R, Sanders B, Ozbaydar M, Lavery K, Warner JJ. Acromioclavicular joint injuries: diagnosis and management. J Am Acad Orthop Surg. 2009 Apr;17(4):207–19)

on the joint ligaments [110–114]. Ice and nonsteroidal anti-inflammatory medications are to be used during this initial immobilization period of approximately 5 days up to 2 weeks to allow for early healing without leading to joint stiffness and loss of motion. Once pain is manageable, the patient is encouraged to initiate early motion as tolerated for restoration of normal mechanics. Scapular stabilization and strengthening exercises are then initiated, with a prolonged period of avoidance of heavy lifting or sports for 2–3 months, to allow for ligamentous scarring and to prevent progression to a Type III injury [112, 115].

For acute Type III injuries, rehabilitation was shown in many studies to result in equal functional outcomes when compared to surgical treatment. Non-operative management was also associated with fewer complications, particularly in comparison to surgical intervention and improved outcomes [116–119]. A recent review of the literature, by Beitzel et al., regarding management of acromioclavicular dislocations compared non-operative to operative management, showing similarly favorable clinical outcomes (88% operatively managed and 85.5% non-operatively managed) despite more anatomic reductions (59%) seen with operative versus non-operative (14.7%). Return to sport, as well as return to work, was also observed to be quicker in the non-operative patients who needed approximately half the recovery time as operatively managed patients in the literature review [110]. However, non-operative management for Type III injuries remains controversial with some recent literature stating that non-operative management leads to a higher prevalence of scapular dyskinesia and symptoms of "SICK" (Scapular malposition, Inferior medial border prominence, Coracoid pain and malposition, and dysKinesis) scapula [120]. Furthermore, there are numerous studies that document potential sequelae of non-operative therapy in Type I and II injuries, and patients should be aware of the possibility of persistent symptoms, including the potential development of posttraumatic AC joint arthritis. A series of studies documented a range of minor symptoms including clicking or pain with shoulder-stressing activity to more major symptoms of persistent pain and loss of function requiring eventual surgical intervention at varying rates with non-operative management [117, 121, 122]. Most athletes and laborers, however, are able to achieve an appropriate level of strength and function to return to sport and profession with adequate rehabilitation attempts [105, 107, 110, 123, 124]. However, there may be an indication for early operative management in aging athletes if the initial injury is severe and if continued symptoms prevent his or her return to the desired level of activity.

If there is persistent pain or degenerative changes, an AC joint corticosteroid injection may be considered as an effective adjuvant treatment. Recent literature regarding the use of ultrasound for injection showed significant improvement in injection success rate in terms of steroid localization [125–127]. A study by Edelson et al. showed a 6-month improvement in patient outcomes with the use of injection for isolated AC disease. However, outcomes were significantly worse in patients with accompanying shoulder pathology [125]. The use of ultrasound is increasing and may lead to an increased rate of intra-articular penetration. While intra-articular injections have been found to be significantly superior in reducing pain with crossover arm test, a recent study reported similar improvements in VAS pain, pain at night, and pain on crossover arm test with a peri-articular AC joint injection at up to 3 weeks after injection [128].

Many studies have shown to highlight the effectiveness of steroid injections for isolated, AC joint pathology as both diagnostic and therapeutic [129–131]. Hossain et al. evaluated the use of injection in patients with primary acromioclavicular arthritis and found it to be an effective treatment, with improvement documented for approximately 12 months and benefit up to 5 years. Important for the aging athlete, this study also reported that injections were more effective in the younger patients, and pain relief tended to diminish over long-term use [132].

Operative Management and Return to Sport

For end-stage degenerative changes, or persistent mechanical symptoms despite conservative treatment, an open or arthroscopic Mumford procedure (distal clavicle resection) is a valid option for an aging athlete with a stable AC joint [133–136]. Resection surgery of an unstable joint may lead to worsening symptoms of instability [107, 131]. For AC joint instability, there is a relative consensus regarding operative management of Type IV–VI injuries due to the morbidity and loss of function associated with these injuries and chronic insult to neighboring soft tissue structures [107, 110]. Type III injuries that have failed a long course of conservative treatment may also be considered for surgical intervention. There is no well-defined, gold standard operative technique or defined timeframe for surgery. A recent review conducted by Beitzel et al. demonstrated a general consensus that operative management is warranted for Type IV–VI lesions; however, they found poorly defined conclusions from studies evaluating early versus delayed operative intervention or anatomic versus nonanatomic surgical reconstruction techniques [110]. Although there are numerous techniques for surgery, the general goals of an operative procedure can be divided into (1) primary AC joint fixation, (2) fixation between coracoid process and clavicle, and (3) ligament reconstruction [107]. No consensus in the literature exists regarding optimal surgical technique, but most agree that anatomic reduction is preferred and ligamentous supplementation is necessary for successful outcome [137–140].

Anatomic restoration was also shown to be biomechanically advantageous [141]. This chapter does not go into the subtleties of each various technique, but knowledge of each is necessary as the operative complications are directly related to the hardware, biologic material, and technique involved. These complications include loss of joint reduction, pin migration, as well as coracoid and clavicle fracture [142]. A recent study reported an overall complication rate of 27.1% (16/59) with cortical fixation buttons or tendon grafts for anatomic coracoclavicular ligament reconstruction. Satisfactory repair was reported at 83.2% at 24 months [143]. The most frequent complications reported in this group include coracoid fracture, clavicle fracture, graft rupture, and hardware failure. Assuming successful surgery without major complication, favorable outcomes were observed in the operative population, especially considering the initial higher severity of injury. There is, however, no well-defined evidence for the aging athlete and functional outcomes regarding sport status after surgery, though numerous studies report a longer recovery time and delay in return to sport (or work) with operative management [137].

Results for one specific type of fixed reconstruction for Type III–IV injuries, using the AC-hook plate, report "good" and "very good" outcomes in 84% of patients regarding pain relief and 89% "excellent" and "good" results regarding functional outcome [144]. These results appear to be relatively consistent across the literature for all different techniques, but the nonstandardized surgical techniques and indications for surgery make generalization difficult, and generalizing these outcomes for the aging athlete population is even more challenging. It is also important to note that, to date, there are no high-quality, randomized, prospective studies evaluating non-operative versus operative treatment, even with situations of "agreed upon" operative indications and that the nonuniformity of surgical technique and indications makes a meta-analysis of the current literature nearly impossible [115]. Further research is needed regarding the optimal surgical intervention, technique, timing, and return to sport, particularly, for the aging athlete.

Conclusion

Acromioclavicular dislocations are most commonly classified using the Rockwood classification, with Type I–II injury as an indication for non-operative management and

Type IV–VI as an indication for operative management. Type III injuries are controversial in the literature. The current evidence appears to support initial management with non-operative treatment given the lower complication rates and faster return to sport and/or work. Failure of conservative measures, chronic pain or instability, and loss of strength/function in the affected extremity during sport or laboring may be indications for operative management. The development of future studies, with standardized surgical technique and a focus on functional outcome and return to sport, is imperative for the optimal management of AC joint injuries in the aging athletic population.

Glenohumeral Arthritis in the Aging Athlete

Introduction

Osteoarthritis (OA) is the most frequent cause of disability in the United States and the most common degenerative pathology in the shoulder joint. This can be debilitating for the aging athlete population. Primary glenohumeral osteoarthritis is present in approximately 2–5% of all shoulder pain complaints [145], with shoulder pain a presenting complaint in up to 21% of adults in the US and Western countries [146–148]. Intervention for glenohumeral osteoarthritis is dependent upon multiple patient factors: age, the presence of concomitant diagnoses, and activity level are important considerations for the successful management of this condition. In the aging, less active population, the options for management of end-stage disease are growing, and the success of arthroplasty has made joint replacement a very attractive option. Regarding the aging athlete population, a balance must be made between management of symptoms while preserving activity level and return to sport. In this section, we will discuss the evaluation of the aging athlete with glenohumeral arthritis, the complexities of each presentation, and what treatment options may help to achieve the best functional outcome.

Patient Evaluation

As with the other conditions discussed, evaluation of the patient starts with the history and physical examination. Important facets of the patient history include activity level, functional expectations, comorbidities, sports, occupation, and hobbies. These factors may dictate treatment options and help to predict long-term outcome. History of systemic rheumatologic disease or past trauma to the glenohumeral joint should be addressed, as these will also play a significant role in the management. Studies indicate that younger patients (those less than 60 years old) with OA are more likely to have experienced prior trauma with one-sided joint degeneration [149]. A recent study by Saltzman et al. demonstrated that primary osteoarthritis was present in only 21% of patients under the age of 50, compared with 66% of those older than 50 [150]. Younger patients had much more complex histories, including diagnoses of capsulorrhaphy arthropathy, posttraumatic arthritis, osteonecrosis, and rheumatoid arthritis. This information is important to collect in the history, prior to examination and radiographs. The typical presenting symptoms consist of progressive pain, stiffness, and loss of motion and strength.

Radiographic assessment should include a true anteroposterior view and axillary view. Typical findings include loss of glenohumeral joint space, glenoid and humeral subchondral sclerosis, osteophytes typically at the inferior humeral head, and bone cysts near the subchondral surface (Fig. 10.9). Close attention should be paid to the amount of glenoid bone loss, which is almost always posterior, as this has significant implications for shoulder arthroplasty. Glenoid retroversion is first assessed on an axillary

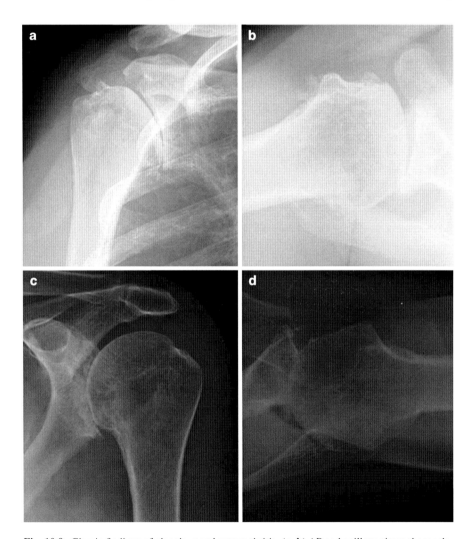

Fig. 10.9 Classic findings of glenohumeral osteoarthritis. (**a, b**) AP and axillary views show sclerosis, narrowing, and mild retroversion with a posterior wear pattern. (**c, d**) Severe osteoarthritis, with sclerosis, narrowing, osteophyte formation, and severe posterior eccentric wear pattern (biconcave glenoid)

radiograph and better visualized for formal calculation using a computed tomography (CT) scan [151]. Retroversion, humeral head posterior subluxation, eccentric glenoid wear, or deficient glenoid bone stock can be assessed on these images (Fig. 10.10). The Walch classification is often used to assess for concentric versus eccentric glenoid wear patterns, the presence of biconcavity, and the degree of glenoid bone loss (Fig. 10.11). These findings are significant, as studies showed that nonconcentric or posteriorly eroded glenoids with severe retroversion have less predictable functional improvement after arthroplasty than patients without the recognized deficiency [152, 153].

Non-operative Management and Return to Sport

For the aging athlete with glenohumeral osteoarthritis, a trial of non-operative therapy—especially for patients with mild-to-moderate OA—is usually warranted [154, 155]. Short-term lifestyle and occupational modifications may be necessary and can be effective when used in combination with pain management and gentle physical therapy. Physical therapy regimens generally focus on range of motion, as well as isometric strengthening of the rotator cuff and scapulothoracic musculature [156]. Intra-articular steroid injections, in combination with nonnarcotic pain regimens, were shown to be effective for pain relief though it is recommended that no more than three corticosteroid injections be placed into a single glenohumeral joint [154,

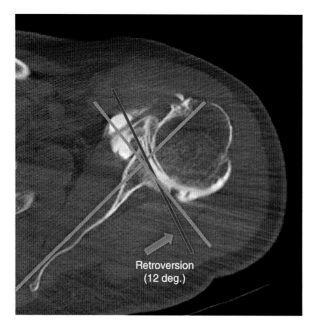

Fig. 10.10 *Glenoid retroversion:* Friedman method of calculating glenoid retroversion for glenohumeral osteoarthritis (Friedman et al., 1992). The extent (approximately 12° of retroversion) and pattern of bone erosion are shown

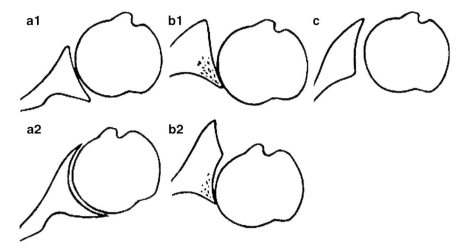

Fig. 10.11 Walch classification for glenoid wear patterns with osteoarthritis of the glenohumeral joint (From: P. Habermeyer, PhD; P. Magosch, MD; V. Luz ; S. Lichtenberg, MD, Three-Dimensional Glenoid Deformity in Patients with Osteoarthritis: A Radiographic Analysis J Bone Joint Surg Am, 2006 Jun;88(6):1301–1307)

157]. The use of viscosupplementation is reported but without strong evidence for use in the non-operative treatment of shoulder osteoarthritis.

Though non-operative treatment reduces the risks and immediate loss of activity common with operative intervention, persistent and progressive glenoid bone erosion may be a significant contraindication to non-operative management [154]. Worsening pain and loss of motion in this cohort are correlated with progressive glenoid erosion, and delay of operative management in these patients may lead to a procedure that cannot be performed in one step alone; it may require osseous augmentation and grafting prior to arthroplasty. Increasing complexity of the procedure is often associated with greater surgical complications and less predictable outcomes.

To date, virtually no literature exists regarding return to sport following non-operative treatment for glenohumeral osteoarthritis. Return to sport will invariably be related to the level of activity of the patient and the specific type of sport played (i.e., golf, swimming, tennis, etc.). Hence, further evidence is required regarding the optimal nonsurgical management for the aging athlete.

Operative Management and Return to Sport

With failure of non-operative measures, surgery is usually indicated for pain relief and functional restoration. The primary procedures offered to patients include arthroscopic debridement with or without capsular release and arthroplasty options such as total shoulder replacement, hemiarthroplasty, humeral head resurfacing, and reverse total shoulder arthroplasty. Arthroscopic joint debridement, with or without release of the GH capsule, was used as a means to increase range of motion and achieve pain relief.

However, recent reviews revealed a paucity of high-quality evidence to recommend arthroscopic debridement as an effective pre-adjunct to arthroplasty for younger, more active individuals. Some evidence suggests improvement in pain relief and short-term patient satisfaction [158, 159], while some reviews report that microfracture and capsular release may also be effective for joint preservation [160]. Biologic techniques for joint preservation such as autologous chondrocyte implantation, osteochondral allografts, and soft tissue interposition arthroplasties have been described, mostly for younger patients. While initially promising [161], most studies were unable to reproduce the initial success observed with biologics [162–165]. In short, higher-quality evidence is warranted before these newer therapies can be recommended as a reliable alternative to arthroplasty, particularly for younger subsets of aging athletes.

Total shoulder arthroplasty (TSA)was shown in multiple studies to be the most favorable procedure with the most predictable outcomes for advanced glenohumeral arthritis (Fig. 10.12). In comparison to hemiarthroplasty, despite the theoretical advantages of avoiding glenoid components, TSA was shown to provide better functional outcome with less likelihood of revision than hemiarthroplasty [166]. However, it has also been stated that due to a poor understanding of the complications and natural history of each procedure (i.e., continued glenoid erosion versus glenoid component loosening), additional higher-level studies with longer follow-up are necessary to better compare these techniques [166].

The success rates for arthroplasty in younger individuals tend to be worse than those in the older cohorts. Though complex in etiology, this is likely due to secondary arthritis diagnoses and concomitant shoulder pathology combined with continuity of more active lifestyles. A review by Denard et al. reported that diagnoses of capsulorrhaphy arthropathy, posttraumatic arthritis, and rheumatoid arthritis, which were most common in younger patients, were associated with higher residual functional deficits at the time of final follow-up with higher complication rates [154, 167].

In an older subset of aging athletes, several studies reported successful return to sport after arthroplasty. A study by McCarty et al. found that 71% of patients ($n = 75$ patients, $n = 86$ arthroplasties, mean age = 65.5 years old at follow-up) had an improvement in their ability to play their sport, with swimming, tennis, and golf the most favorable improvement including full return to sport. The mean time for return to sport was approximately 3.6 months until return and 5.8 months until full participation [168]. A more recent study demonstrated that patients with a mean age of 71 years old (range, 33–88) at the time of surgery, who underwent a TSA had a return to sports rate of 100% if they were active in that sporting activity prior to surgery [169]. Swimming was the most popular sport in this cohort, but no conclusions were made regarding postoperative function compared to preoperative level. In a recent survey study ($n = 35$), 31 of 35 (89%) golfers were able to return to golf following TSA with an average time of 8.4 months needed to return to sport. Additionally, authors found a statistically significant increase in driving distance and a significant improvement in handicap after surgery [170].

Overall, the literature strongly supports the use of TSA for relief of pain, restoration of function, and return to sport in older, active patients. However, the optimal treatment for the younger, aging athlete, particularly those who continue to place significant high demands on their shoulders remains controversial. Many surgeons

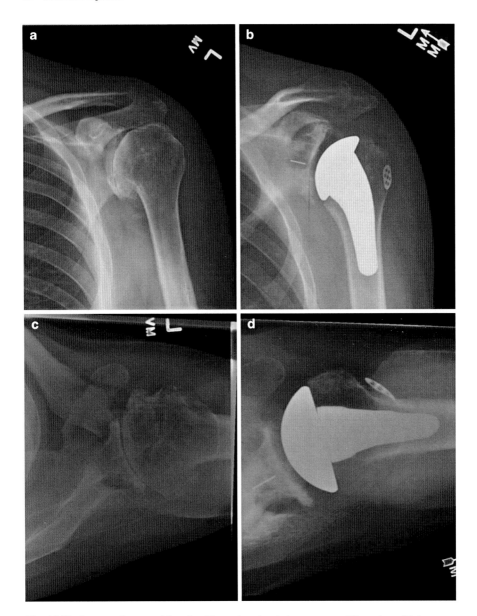

Fig. 10.12 Preoperative true AP and axillary view (**a**, **c**) demonstrate obliteration of joint space and inferior osteophyte formation consistent with severe osteoarthritis. Postoperative true AP and axillary view (**b**, **d**) provide good visualization of a total shoulder prosthesis with restoration of the glenohumeral joint space

advocate treatment with other techniques, including humeral resurfacing, hemiarthroplasty with or without glenoid "ream-and-run," or biologic alternatives; however, these were not borne out of the current literature at this time. The theory for resurfacing or humeral head replacement without glenoid component implantation focuses on removing the risk of glenoid loosening which was found to be present in up to one-third of anatomic total shoulder arthroplasties at 10 years (Fig. 10.13).

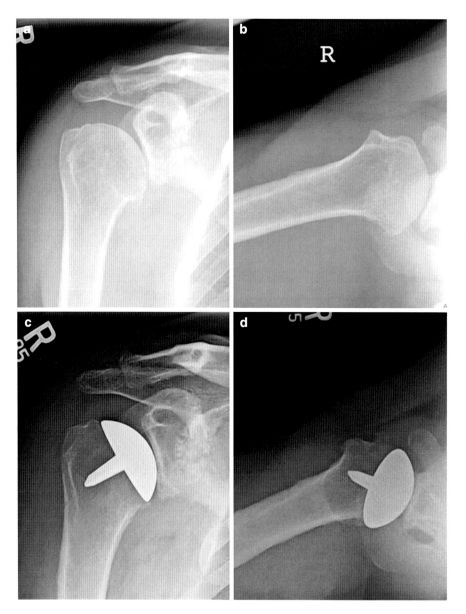

Fig. 10.13 A 40-year-old male heavy laborer with severe osteoarthritis, demonstrated on AP and axillary view (**a**, **b**). Due to concerns of early glenoid component loosening, humeral head resurfacing was performed rather than total shoulder arthroplasty (**c**, **d**)

More studies, with longer follow-up and close evaluation of the athletic participation, are necessary to draw conclusions regarding the optimal treatment for the younger, aging athlete population.

Conclusion

Osteoarthritis is the most common degenerative process in the shoulder and can be associated with significant pain and loss of function. The majority of cases are primary osteoarthritis in the older cohorts of aging athletes. Younger cohorts will more commonly present with secondary arthritis. Common presentations for both cohorts are progressive pain and loss of motion leading to severe activity impairment. A thorough patient history and radiographic evaluation is essential for determining the best treatment option. Non-operative management is usually the initial mainstay of treatment. For end-stage disease, total shoulder arthroplasty is a successful option, particularly for the older, aging athlete. Optimal management of the younger, aging athlete remains a challenge. Further studies for this ever-increasing cohort are needed to assess for surgical alternatives that will prolong participation in athletic activity without significant risk of complication.

References

1. Knesek M, Skendzel JG, Dines JS, Altchek DW, Allen AA, Bedi A. Diagnosis and management of superior labral anterior posterior tears in throwing athletes. Am J Sports Med. 2013;41(2):444–60.
2. Aydin N, Sirin E, Arya A. Superior labrum anterior to posterior lesions of the shoulder: diagnosis and arthroscopic management. World J Orthop. 2014;5(3):344–50.
3. Manske R, Ellenbecker T. Current concepts in shoulder examination of the overhead athlete. Int J Sports Phys Ther. 2013;8(5):554–78.
4. Michener LA, Doukas WC, Murphy KP, Walsworth MK. Diagnostic accuracy of history and physical examination of superior labrum anterior-posterior lesions. J Athl Train. 2011;46(4):343–8.
5. O'Brien SJ, Pagnani MJ, Fealy S, McGlynn SR, Wilson JB. The active compression test: a new and effective test for diagnosing labral tears and acromioclavicular joint abnormality. Am J Sports Med. 1998;26(5):610–3.
6. Parentis MA, Glousman RE, Mohr KS, Yocum LA. An evaluation of the provocative tests for superior labral anterior posterior lesions. Am J Sports Med. 2006;34(2):265–8.
7. Keener JD, Brophy RH. Superior labral tears of the shoulder: pathogenesis, evaluation, and treatment. J Am Acad Orthop Surg. 2009;17(10):627–37.
8. Jee WH, McCauley TR, Katz LD, Matheny JM, Ruwe PA, Daigneault JP. Superior labral anterior posterior (SLAP) lesions of the glenoid labrum: reliability and accuracy of MR arthrography for diagnosis. Radiology. 2001;218(1):127–32.
9. Connor PM, Banks DM, Tyson AB, Coumas JS, D'Alessandro DF. Magnetic resonance imaging of the asymptomatic shoulder of overhead athletes: a 5-year follow-up study. Am J Sports Med. 2003;31(5):724–7.
10. Bedi A, Allen AA. Superior labral lesions anterior to posterior-evaluation and arthroscopic management. Clin Sports Med. 2008;27(4):607–30.

11. Edwards SL, Lee JA, Bell JE, Packer JD, Ahmad CS, Levine WN, Bigliani LU, Blaine TA. Nonoperative treatment of superior labrum anterior posterior tears: improvements in pain, function, and quality of life. Am J Sports Med. 2010;38(7):1456–61.
12. Morgan CD, Burkhart SS, Palmeri M, Gillespie M. Type II SLAP lesions: three subtypes and their relationships to superior instability and rotator cuff tears. Arthroscopy. 1998;14(6):553–65.
13. Erickson J, Lavery K, Monica J, Gatt C, Dhawan A. Surgical treatment of symptomatic superior labrum anterior-posterior tears in patients older than 40 years: a systematic review. Am J Sports Med. 2015;43:1274–82.
14. Boileau P, Parratte S, Chuinard C, Roussanne Y, Shia D, Bicknell R. Arthroscopic treatment of isolated type II SLAP lesions: biceps tenodesis as an alternative to reinsertion. Am J Sports Med. 2009;37(5):929–36.
15. Neuman BJ, Boisvert CB, Reiter B, Lawson K, Ciccotti MG, Cohen SB. Results of arthroscopic repair of type II superior labral anterior posterior lesions in overhead athletes: assessment of return to preinjury playing level and satisfaction. Am J Sports Med. 2011;39(9):1883–8.
16. Provencher MT, McCormick F, Dewing C, McIntire S, Solomon D. A prospective analysis of 179 type 2 superior labrum anterior and posterior repairs: outcomes and factors associated with success and failure. Am J Sports Med. 2013;41(4):880–6.
17. Denard PJ, Lädermann A, Parsley BK, Burkhart SS. Arthroscopic biceps tenodesis compared with repair of isolated type II SLAP lesions in patients older than 35 years. Orthopedics. 2014;37(3):e292–7.
18. Ek ET, Shi LL, Tompson JD, Freehill MT, Warner JJ. Surgical treatment of isolated type II superior labrum anterior-posterior (SLAP) lesions: repair versus biceps tenodesis. J Shoulder Elbow Surg. 2014;23(7):1059–65.
19. Kim SJ, Lee IS, Kim SH, Woo CM, Chun YM. Arthroscopic repair of concomitant type II SLAP lesions in large to massive rotator cuff tears: comparison with biceps tenotomy. Am J Sports Med. 2012;40(12):2786–93.
20. Abbot AE, Li X, Busconi BD. Arthroscopic treatment of concomitant superior labral anterior posterior (SLAP) lesions and rotator cuff tears in patients over the age of 45 years. Am J Sports Med. 2009;37(7):1358–62.
21. Voos JE, Pearle AD, Mattern CJ, Cordasco FA, Allen AA, Warren RF. Outcomes of combined arthroscopic rotator cuff and labral repair. Am J Sports Med. 2007;35(7):1174–9. Epub 2007 Mar 26
22. Werner BC, Brockmeier SF, Miller MD. Etiology, diagnosis, and management of failed SLAP repair. J Am Acad Orthop Surg. 2014;22(9):554–65.
23. Franceschi F, Longo UG, Ruzzini L, Rizzello G, Maffulli N, Denaro V. No advantages in repairing a type II superior labrum anterior and posterior (SLAP) lesion when associated with rotator cuff repair in patients over age 50: a randomized controlled trial. Am J Sports Med. 2008;36(2):247–53.
24. Zhang AL, Kreulen C, Ngo SS, Hame SL, Wang JC, Gamradt SC. Demographic trends in arthroscopic SLAP repair in the United States. Am J Sports Med. 2012;40(5):1144–7.
25. Patterson BM, Creighton RA, Spang JT, Roberson JR, Kamath GV. Surgical trends in the treatment of superior labrum anterior and posterior lesions of the shoulder: analysis of data from the American Board of Orthopaedic Surgery Certification Examination Database. Am J Sports Med. 2014;42(8):1904–10.
26. Egol KA, Koval KJ, Zuckerman JD. Handbook of fracture. 4th ed. Philadelphia: Lippincott Williams & Wilkins; 2010.
27. Zacchilli MA, Owens BD. Epidemiology of shoulder dislocations presenting to emergency departments in the United States. J Bone Joint Surg Am. 2010;92(3):542–9.
28. Rowe CR. Prognosis in dislocations of the shoulder. J Bone Joint Surg Am. 1956;38-A(5):957–77.
29. Leroux T, Wasserstein D, Veillette C, Khoshbin A, Henry P, Chahal J, Austin P, Mahomed N, Ogilvie-Harris D. Epidemiology of primary anterior shoulder dislocation requiring closed reduction in Ontario, Canada. Am J Sports Med. 2014;42(2):442–50.

30. Rowe CR, Sakellarides HT. Factors related to recurrences of anterior dislocations of the shoulder. Clin Orthop. 1961;20:40–8.
31. Wheeler JH, Ryan JB, Arciero RA, Molinari RN. Arthroscopic versus nonoperative treatment of acute shoulder dislocations in young athletes. Arthroscopy. 1989;5(3):213–7.
32. te Slaa RL, Brand R, Marti RK. A prospective arthroscopic study of acute first-time anterior shoulder dislocation in the young: a five-year follow-up study. J Shoulder Elbow Surg. 2003;12(6):529–34.
33. McLaughlin HL, MacLellan DI. Recurrent anterior dislocation of the shoulder. II. A comparative study. J Trauma. 1967;7(2):191–201.
34. Neviaser RJ, Neviaser TJ, Neviaser JS. Anterior dislocation of the shoulder and rotator cuff rupture. Clin Orthop Relat Res. 1993;291:103–6.
35. Hawkins RJ, Bell RH, Hawkins RH, Koppert GJ. Anterior dislocation of the shoulder in the older patient. Clin Orthop Relat Res. 1986;206:192–5.
36. Berbig R, Weishaupt D, Prim J, Shahin O. Primary anterior shoulder dislocation and rotator cuff tears. J Shoulder Elbow Surg. 1999;8(3):220–5.
37. Imhoff AB, Ansah P, Tischer T, Reiter C, Bartl C, Hench M, Spang JT, Vogt S. Arthroscopic repair of anterior-inferior glenohumeral instability using a portal at the 5:30-o'clock position: analysis of the effects of age, fixation method, and concomitant shoulder injury on surgical outcomes. Am J Sports Med. 2010;38(9):1795–803.
38. Simank HG, Dauer G, Schneider S, Loew M. Incidence of rotator cuff tears in shoulder dislocations and results of therapy in older patients. Arch Orthop Trauma Surg. 2006;126(4):235–40.
39. Robinson CM, Shur N, Sharpe T, Ray A, Murray IR. Injuries associated with traumatic anterior glenohumeral dislocations. J Bone Joint Surg Am. 2012;94(1):18–26.
40. Neviaser RJ, Neviaser TJ, Neviaser JS. Concurrent rupture of the rotator cuff and anterior dislocation of the shoulder in the older patient. J Bone Joint Surg Am. 1988;70(9):1308–11.
41. Paxton ES, Dodson CC, Lazarus MD. Shoulder instability in older patients. Orthop Clin North Am. 2014;45(3):377–85.
42. Murthi AM, Ramirez MA. Shoulder dislocation in the older patient. J Am Acad Orthop Surg. 2012;20(10):615–22.
43. Toolanen G, Hildingsson C, Hedlund T, Knibestöl M, Oberg L. Early complications after anterior dislocation of the shoulder in patients over 40 years. An ultrasonographic and electromyographic study. Acta Orthop Scand. 1993;64(5):549–52.
44. Gomberawalla MM, Sekiya JK. Rotator cuff tear and glenohumeral instability: a systematic review. Clin Orthop Relat Res. 2014;472(8):2448–56.
45. Stayner LR, Cummings J, Andersen J, Jobe CM. Shoulder dislocations in patients older than 40 years of age. Orthop Clin North Am. 2000;31:231–9.
46. Porcellini G, Caranzano F, Campi F, Paladini P. Instability and rotator cuff tear. Med Sport Sci. 2012;57:41–52.
47. Porcellini G, Caranzano F, Campi F, Pellegrini A, Paladini P. Glenohumeral instability and rotator cuff tear. Sports Med Arthrosc Rev. 2011;19(4):395–400.
48. Youm T, Takemoto R, Park BK. Acute management of shoulder dislocations. J Am Acad Orthop Surg. 2014;22(12):761–71.
49. Groh GI, Rockwood CA Jr. The terrible triad: anterior dislocation of the shoulder associated with rupture of the rotator cuff and injury to the brachial plexus. J Shoulder Elbow Surg. 1995;4(1 Pt 1):51–3.
50. Pevny T, Hunter RE, Freeman JR. Primary traumatic anterior shoulder dislocation in patients 40 years of age and older. Arthroscopy. 1998;14(3):289–94.
51. Neviaser RJ, Neviaser TJ. Recurrent instability of the shoulder after age 40. J Shoulder Elbow Surg. 1995;4(6):416–8.
52. Porcellini G, Paladini P, Campi F, Paganelli M. Shoulder instability and related rotator cuff tears: arthroscopic findings and treatment in patients aged 40 to 60 years. Arthroscopy. 2006;22(3):270–6.
53. Maier M, Geiger EV, Ilius C, Frank J, Marzi I. Midterm results after operatively stabilised shoulder dislocations in elderly patients. Int Orthop. 2009;33(3):719–23.

54. Shin SJ, Yun YH, Kim DJ, Yoo JD. Treatment of traumatic anterior shoulder dislocation in patients older than 60 years. Am J Sports Med. 2012;40(4):822–7.
55. Yamaguchi K, Ditsios K, Middleton WD, Hildebolt CF, Galatz LM, Teefey SA. The demographic and morphological features of rotator cuff disease. A comparison of asymptomatic and symptomatic shoulders. J Bone Joint Surg Am. 2006;88(8):1699–704.
56. Armstrong A. Evaluation and management of adult shoulder pain: a focus on rotator cuff disorders, acromioclavicular joint arthritis, and glenohumeral arthritis. Med Clin North Am. 2014;98(4):755–75, xii.
57. Fukuda H. The management of partial-thickness tears of the rotator cuff. J Bone Joint Surg Br. 2003;85(1):3–11.
58. Hurschler C, Wülker N, Windhagen H, Hellmers N, Plumhoff P. Evaluation of the lag sign tests for external rotator function of the shoulder. J Shoulder Elbow Surg. 2004;13(3):298–304.
59. Hertel R, Ballmer FT, Lombert SM, Gerber C. Lag signs in the diagnosis of rotator cuff rupture. J Shoulder Elbow Surg. 1996;5(4):307–13.
60. MacDonald PB, Clark P, Sutherland K. An analysis of the diagnostic accuracy of the Hawkins and Neer subacromial impingement signs. J Shoulder Elbow Surg. 2000;9(4):299–301.
61. Hermans J, Luime JJ, Meuffels DE, Reijman M, Simel DL, Bierma-Zeinstra SM. Does this patient with shoulder pain have rotator cuff disease?: The Rational Clinical Examination systematic review. JAMA. 2013;310(8):837–47.
62. Bigliani LU, Morrison DS, April EW. The morphology of the acromion and its relationship to rotator cuff tears. Orthop Trans. 1986;10:228.
63. Chahal J, Mall N, MacDonald PB, Van Thiel G, Cole BJ, Romeo AA, Verma NN. The role of subacromial decompression in patients undergoing arthroscopic repair of full-thickness tears of the rotator cuff: a systematic review and meta-analysis. Arthroscopy. 2012;28(5):720–7.
64. Lenza M, Buchbinder R, Takwoingi Y, Johnston RV, Hanchard NC, Faloppa F. Magnetic resonance imaging, magnetic resonance arthrography and ultrasonography for assessing rotator cuff tears in people with shoulder pain for whom surgery is being considered. Cochrane Database Syst Rev. 2013;(24):9.
65. Iannotti JP, Ciccone J, Buss DD, Visotsky JL, Mascha E, Cotman K, Rawool NM. Accuracy of office-based ultrasonography of the shoulder for the diagnosis of rotator cuff tears. J Bone Joint Surg Am. 2005;87(6):1305–11.
66. Wolff AB, Sethi P, Sutton KM, Covey AS, Magit DP, Medvecky M. Partial-thickness rotator cuff tears. J Am Acad Orthop Surg. 2006;14(13):715–25.
67. Rhon DI, Boyles RB, Cleland JA. One-year outcome of subacromial corticosteroid injection compared with manual physical therapy for the management of the unilateral shoulder impingement syndrome: a pragmatic randomized trial. Ann Intern Med. 2014;161(3):161–9.
68. Yamaguchi K, Tetro AM, Blam O, Evanoff BA, Teefey SA, Middleton WD. Natural history of asymptomatic rotator cuff tears: a longitudinal analysis of asymptomatic tears detected sonographically. J Shoulder Elbow Surg. 2001;10(3):199–203.
69. Moosmayer S, Tariq R, Stiris M, Smith HJ. The natural history of asymptomatic rotator cuff tears: a three-year follow-up of fifty cases. J Bone Joint Surg Am. 2013;95(14):1249–55.
70. Maman E, Harris C, White L, Tomlinson G, Shashank M, Boynton E. Outcome of nonoperative treatment of symptomatic rotator cuff tears monitored by magnetic resonance imaging. J Bone Joint Surg Am. 2009;91(8):1898–906.
71. Safran O, Schroeder J, Bloom R, Weil Y, Milgrom C. Natural history of nonoperatively treated symptomatic rotator cuff tears in patients 60 years old or younger. Am J Sports Med. 2011;39(4):710–4.
72. Zingg PO, Jost B, Sukthankar A, Buhler M, Pfirrmann CW, Gerber C. Clinical and structural outcomes of nonoperative management of massive rotator cuff tears. J Bone Joint Surg Am. 2007;89(9):1928–34.
73. Moosmayer S, Lund G, Seljom US, Haldorsen B, Svege IC, Hennig T, Pripp AH, Smith HJ. Tendon repair compared with physiotherapy in the treatment of rotator cuff tears: a randomized controlled study in 103 cases with a five-year follow-up. J Bone Joint Surg Am. 2014;96(18):1504–14.

74. Fucentese SF, von Roll AL, Pfirrmann CW, Gerber C, Jost B. Evolution of nonoperatively treated symptomatic isolated full-thickness supraspinatus tears. J Bone Joint Surg Am. 2012;94(9):801–8.
75. Attiq-ur-Rehman, Wajid MA, Ahmad T. Shoulder impingement syndrome: outcome of arthroscopic subacromial decompression. J Coll Physicians Surg Pak. 2009;19(10):636–9.
76. Biberthaler P, Beirer M, Kirchhoff S, Braunstein V, Wiedemann E, Kirchhoff C. Significant benefit for older patients after arthroscopic subacromial decompression: a long-term follow-up study. Int Orthop. 2013;37(3):457–62.
77. Patel VR, Singh D, Calvert PT, Bayley JI. Arthroscopic subacromial decompression: results and factors affecting outcome. J Shoulder Elbow Surg. 1999;8(3):231–7.
78. Soyer J, Vaz S, Pries P, Clarac JP. The relationship between clinical outcomes and the amount of arthroscopic acromial resection. Arthroscopy. 2003;19(1):34–9.
79. Klintberg IH, Svantesson U, Karlsson J. Long-term patient satisfaction and functional outcome 8-11 years after subacromial decompression. Knee Surg Sports Traumatol Arthrosc. 2010;18(3):394–403.
80. Saltychev M, Aärimaa V, Virolainen P, Laimi K. Conservative treatment or surgery for shoulder impingement: systematic review and meta-analysis. Disabil Rehabil. 2015;37:1–8.
81. Dorrestijn O, Stevens M, Winters JC, van der Meer K, Diercks RL. Conservative or surgical treatment for subacromial impingement syndrome? A systematic review. J Shoulder Elbow Surg. 2009;18(4):652–60.
82. Pedowitz RA, Yamaguchi K, Ahmad CS, Burks RT, Flatow EL, Green A, Wies JL, St Andre J, Boyer K, Iannotti JP, Miller BS, Tashjian R, Watters WC III, Weber K, Turkelson CM, Raymond L, Sluka P, McGowan R. American Academy of Orthopaedic Surgeons Clinical Practice Guideline on: optimizing the management of rotator cuff problems. J Bone Joint Surg Am. 2012;94(2):163–7.
83. Mall NA, Kim HM, Keener JD, Steger-May K, Teefey SA, Middleton WD, Stobbs G, Yamaguchi K. Symptomatic progression of asymptomatic rotator cuff tears: a prospective study of clinical and sonographic variables. J Bone Joint Surg Am. 2010;92(16):2623–33.
84. Cole BJ, LP MC III, Kang RW, Alford W, Lewis PB, Hayden JK. Arthroscopic rotator cuff repair: prospective functional outcome and repair integrity at minimum 2-year follow-up. J Shoulder Elbow Surg. 2007;16(5):579–85.
85. Paxton ES, Teefey SA, Dahiya N, Keener JD, Yamaguchi K, Galatz LM. Clinical and radiographic outcomes of failed repairs of large or massive rotator cuff tears: minimum ten-year follow-up. J Bone Joint Surg Am. 2013;95(7):627–32.
86. Shin SJ. A comparison of 2 repair techniques for partial-thickness articular-sided rotator cuff tears. Arthroscopy. 2012;28(1):25–33.
87. Ide J, Maeda S, Takagi K. A comparison of arthroscopic and open rotator cuff repair. Arthroscopy. 2005;21(9):1090–8.
88. Morse K, Davis AD, Afra R, Kaye EK, Schepsis A, Voloshin I. Arthroscopic versus mini-open rotator cuff repair: a comprehensive review and meta-analysis. Am J Sports Med. 2008;36(9):1824–8.
89. Bishop J, Klepps S, Lo IK, Bird J, Gladstone JN, Flatow EL. Cuff integrity after arthroscopic versus open rotator cuff repair: a prospective study. J Shoulder Elbow Surg. 2006;15(3):290–9.
90. Apreleva M, Ozbaydar M, Fitzgibbons PG, Warner JJ. Rotator cuff tears: the effect of the reconstruction method on three-dimensional repair site area. Arthroscopy. 2002;18(5):519–26.
91. Ahmad CS, Stewart AM, Izquierdo R, Bigliani LU. Tendon-bone interface motion in transosseous suture and suture anchor rotator cuff repair techniques. Am J Sports Med. 2005;33(11):1667–71.
92. Saridakis P, Jones G. Outcomes of single-row and double-row arthroscopic rotator cuff repair: a systematic review. J Bone Joint Surg Am. 2010;92(3):732–42.
93. Mihata T, Watanabe C, Fukunishi K, Ohue M, Tsujimura T, Fujiwara K, Kinoshita M. Functional and structural outcomes of single-row versus double-row versus combined double-row and suture-bridge repair for rotator cuff tears. Am J Sports Med. 2011;39(10):2091–8.

94. Duquin TR, Buyea C, Bisson LJ. Which method of rotator cuff repair leads to the highest rate of structural healing? A systematic review. Am J Sports Med. 2010;38(4):835–41.
95. DeHaan AM, Axelrad TW, Kaye E, Silvestri L, Puskas B, Foster TE. Does double-row rotator cuff repair improve functional outcome of patients compared with single-row technique? A systematic review. Am J Sports Med. 2012;40(5):1176–85.
96. McCormick F, Gupta A, Bruce B, Harris J, Abrams G, Wilson H, Hussey K, Cole BJ. Single-row, double-row, and transosseous equivalent techniques for isolated supraspinatus tendon tears with minimal atrophy: a retrospective comparative outcome and radiographic analysis at minimum 2-year followup. Int J Shoulder Surg. 2014;8(1):15–20.
97. Ji X, Bi C, Wang F, Wang Q. Arthroscopic versus mini-open rotator cuff repair: an up-to-date meta-analysis of randomized controlled trials. Arthroscopy. 2015;31(1):118–24.
98. Kim YS, Chung SW, Kim JY, Ok JH, Park I, Oh JH. Is early passive motion exercise necessary after arthroscopic rotator cuff repair? Am J Sports Med. 2012;40(4):815–21.
99. Chang KV, Hung CY, Han DS, Chen WS, Wang TG, Chien KL. Early versus delayed passive range of motion exercise for arthroscopic rotator cuff repair: a meta-analysis of randomized controlled trials. Am J Sports Med. 2015;43:1265–73.
100. Chan K, MacDermid JC, Hoppe DJ, Ayeni OR, Bhandari M, Foote CJ, Athwal GS. Delayed versus early motion after arthroscopic rotator cuff repair: a meta-analysis. J Shoulder Elbow Surg. 2014;23(11):1631–9.
101. Bassett RW, Cofield RH. Acute tears of the rotator cuff. The timing of surgical repair. Clin Orthop Relat Res. 1983;175:18–24.
102. Lähteenmäki HE, Virolainen P, Hiltunen A, Heikkilä J, Nelimarkka OI. Results of early operative treatment of rotator cuff tears with acute symptoms. J Shoulder Elbow Surg. 2006;15(2):148–53.
103. Mukovozov I, Byun S, Farrokhyar F, Wong I. Time to surgery in acute rotator cuff tear: a systematic review. Bone Joint Res. 2013;2(7):122–8.
104. Kaplan LD, Flanigan DC, Norwig J, Jost P, Bradley J. Prevalence and variance of shoulder injuries in elite collegiate football players. Am J Sports Med. 2005;33(8):1142–6.
105. Bradley JP, Elkousy H. Decision making: operative versus nonoperative treatment of acromioclavicular joint injuries. Clin Sports Med. 2003;22(2):277–90.
106. Babhulkar A, Pawaskar A. Acromioclavicular joint dislocations. Curr Rev Musculoskelet Med. 2014;7(1):33–9.
107. Simovitch R, Sanders B, Ozbaydar M, Lavery K, Warner JJ. Acromioclavicular joint injuries: diagnosis and management. J Am Acad Orthop Surg. 2009;17(4):207–19.
108. Tauber M. Management of acute acromioclavicular joint dislocations: current concepts. Arch Orthop Trauma Surg. 2013;133(7):985–95.
109. Cox JS. Current method of treatment of acromioclavicular joint dislocations. Orthopedics. 1992;15(9):1041–4.
110. Beitzel K, Cote MP, Apostolakos J, Solovyova O, Judson CH, Ziegler CG, Edgar CM, Imhoff AB, Arciero RA, Mazzocca AD. Current concepts in the treatment of acromioclavicular joint dislocations. Arthroscopy. 2013;29(2):387–97.
111. Lemos MJ. The evaluation and treatment of the injured acromioclavicular joint in athletes. Am J Sports Med. 1998;26(1):137–44.
112. Mazzocca AD, Arciero RA, Bicos J. Evaluation and treatment of acromioclavicular joint injuries. Am J Sports Med. 2007;35(2):316–29.
113. Cote MP, Wojcik KE, Gomlinski G, Mazzocca AD. Rehabilitation of acromioclavicular joint separations: operative and nonoperative considerations. Clin Sports Med. 2010;29(2):213–28.
114. Bontempo NA, Mazzocca AD. Biomechanics and treatment of acromioclavicular and sterno-clavicular joint injuries. Br J Sports Med. 2010;44(5):361–9.
115. Tamaoki MJ, Belloti JC, Lenza M, Matsumoto MH, Gomes Dos Santos JB, Faloppa F. Surgical versus conservative interventions for treating acromioclavicular dislocation of the shoulder in adults. Cochrane Database Syst Rev. 2010;(8):CD007429.
116. Phillips AM, Smart C, Groom AF. Acromioclavicular dislocation: conservative or surgical therapy. Clin Orthop Relat Res. 1998;353:10–7.

117. Bannister GC, Wallace WA, Stableforth PG, Hutson MA. The management of acute acromioclavicular dislocation: a randomised prospective controlled trial. J Bone Joint Surg Br. 1989;71:848–50.
118. Larsen E, Bjerg-Nielsen A, Christensen P. Conservative or surgical treatment of acromioclavicular dislocation. A prospective, controlled, randomized study. J Bone Joint Surg Am. 1986;68(4):552–5.
119. Wojtys EM, Nelson G. Conservative treatment of Grade III acromioclavicular dislocations. Clin Orthop Relat Res. 1991;268:112–9.
120. Murena L, Canton G, Vulcano E, Cherubino P. Scapular dyskinesis and SICK scapula syndrome following surgical treatment of type III acute acromioclavicular dislocations. Knee Surg Sports Traumatol Arthrosc. 2013;21(5):1146–50.
121. Mouhsine E, Garofalo R, Crevoisier X, Farron A. Grade I and II acromioclavicular dislocations: results of conservative treatment. J Shoulder Elbow Surg. 2003;12:599–602.
122. Bergfeld JA, Andrish JT, Clancy WG. Evaluation of the acromioclavicular joint following first- and second-degree sprains. Am J Sports Med. 1978;6:153–9.
123. Walsh WM, Peterson DA, Shelton G, Neumann RD. Shoulder strength following acromioclavicular injury. Am J Sports Med. 1985;13(3):153–8.
124. Glick JM, Milburn LJ, Haggerty JF, Nishimoto D. Dislocated acromioclavicular joint: follow-up study of 35 unreduced acromioclavicular dislocations. Am J Sports Med. 1977;5(6):264–70.
125. Edelson G, Saffuri H, Obid E, Lipovsky E, Ben-David D. Successful injection of the acromioclavicular joint with use of ultrasound: anatomy, technique, and follow-up. J Shoulder Elbow Surg. 2014;23(10):243–50.
126. Borbas P, Kraus T, Clement H, Grechenig S, Weinberg AM, Heidari N. The influence of ultrasound guidance in the rate of success of acromioclavicular joint injection: an experimental study on human cadavers. J Shoulder Elbow Surg. 2012;21(12):1694–7.
127. Daley EL, Bajaj S, Bisson LJ, Cole BJ. Improving injection accuracy of the elbow, knee, and shoulder: does injection site and imaging make a difference? A systematic review. Am J Sports Med. 2011;39(3):656–62.
128. Sabeti-Aschraf M, Stotter C, Thaler C, Kristen K, Schmidt M, Krifter RM, Hexel M, Ostermann R, Hofstaedter T, Graf A, Windhager R. Intra-articular versus periarticular acromioclavicular joint injection: a multicenter, prospective, randomized, controlled trial. Arthroscopy. 2013;29(12):1903–10.
129. Cadet E, Ahmad CS, Levine WN. The management of acromioclavicular joint osteoarthrosis: débride, resect, or leave it alone. Instr Course Lect. 2006;55:75–83.
130. Docimo S Jr, Kornitsky D, Futterman B, Elkowitz DE. Surgical treatment for acromioclavicular joint osteoarthritis: patient selection, surgical options, complications, and outcome. Curr Rev Musculoskelet Med. 2008;1(2):154–60.
131. Shaffer BS. Painful conditions of the acromioclavicular joint. J Am Acad Orthop Surg. 1999;7(3):176–88.
132. Hossain S, Jacobs LG, Hashmi R. The long-term effectiveness of steroid injections in primary acromioclavicular joint arthritis: a five-year prospective study. J Shoulder Elbow Surg. 2008;17(4):535–8.
133. Pensak M, Grumet RC, Slabaugh MA, Bach BR Jr. Open versus arthroscopic distal clavicle resection. Arthroscopy. 2010;26(5):697–704.
134. Elhassan B, Ozbaydar M, Diller D, Massimini D, Higgins LD, Warner JJ. Open versus arthroscopic acromioclavicular joint resection: a retrospective comparison study. Arthroscopy. 2009;25(11):1224–32.
135. Rabalais RD, McCarty E. Surgical treatment of symptomatic acromioclavicular joint problems: a systematic review. Clin Orthop Relat Res. 2007;455:30–7.
136. Charron KM, Schepsis AA, Voloshin I. Arthroscopic distal clavicle resection in athletes: a prospective comparison of the direct and indirect approach. Am J Sports Med. 2007;35(1):53–8.
137. Li X, Ma R, Bedi A, Dines DM, Altchek DW, Dines JS. Management of acromioclavicular joint injuries. J Bone Joint Surg Am. 2014;96(1):73–84. https://doi.org/10.2106/JBJS.L.00734. PubMed PMID: 24382728.

138. Beitzel K, Obopilwe E, Apostolakos J, Cote MP, Russell RP, Charette R, Singh H, Arciero RA, Imhoff AB, Mazzocca AD. Rotational and translational stability of different methods for direct acromioclavicular ligament repair in anatomic acromioclavicular joint reconstruction. Am J Sports Med. 2014;42(9):2141–8.
139. Tauber M, Gordon K, Koller H, Fox M, Resch H. Semitendinosus tendon graft versus a modified Weaver-Dunn procedure for acromioclavicular joint reconstruction in chronic cases: a prospective comparative study. Am J Sports Med. 2009;37(1):181–90.
140. Fraschini G, Ciampi P, Scotti C, Ballis R, Peretti GM. Surgical treatment of chronic acromioclavicular dislocation: comparison between two surgical procedures for anatomic reconstruction. Injury. 2010;41(11):1103–6.
141. Mazzocca AD, Santangelo SA, Johnson ST, Rios CG, Dumonski ML, Arciero RA. A biomechanical evaluation of an anatomical coracoclavicular ligament reconstruction. Am J Sports Med. 2006;34:236–46.
142. Milewski MD, Tompkins M, Giugale JM, Carson EW, Miller MD, Diduch DR. Complications related to anatomic reconstruction of the coracoclavicular ligaments. Am J Sports Med. 2012;40(7):1628–34.
143. Martetschläger F, Horan MP, Warth RJ, Millett PJ. Complications after anatomic fixation and reconstruction of the coracoclavicular ligaments. Am J Sports Med. 2013;41(12):2896–903.
144. Kienast B, Thietje R, Queitsch C, Gille J, Schulz AP, Meiners J. Mid-term results after operative treatment of rockwood grade III-V acromioclavicular joint dislocations with an AC-hook-plate. Eur J Med Res. 2011;16(2):52–6.
145. Meislin RJ, Sperling JW, Stitik TP. Persistent shoulder pain: epidemiology, pathophysiology, and diagnosis. Am J Orthop (Belle Mead NJ). 2005;34(12 Suppl):5–9.
146. Bergenudd H, Lindgärde F, Nilsson B, Petersson CJ. Shoulder pain in middle age. A study of prevalence and relation to occupational work load and psychosocial factors. Clin Orthop Relat Res. 1988;231:234–8.
147. Chakravarty KK, Webley M. Disorders of the shoulder: an often unrecognised cause of disability in elderly people. BMJ. 1990;300(6728):848–9.
148. Chard MD, Hazleman R, Hazleman BL, King RH, Reiss BB. Shoulder disorders in the elderly: a community survey. Arthritis Rheum. 1991;34(6):766–9.
149. Kerr BJ, McCarty EC. Outcome of arthroscopic debridement is worse for patients with glenohumeral arthritis of both sides of the joint. Clin Orthop Relat Res. 2008;466:634–8.
150. Saltzman MD, Mercer DM, Warme WJ, Bertelsen AL, Matsen FA III. Comparison of patients undergoing primary shoulder arthroplasty before and after the age of fifty. J Bone Joint Surg Am. 2010;92:42–7.
151. Friedman RJ, Hawthorne KB, Genez BM. The use of computerized tomography in the measurement of glenoid version. J Bone Joint Surg Am. 1992;74(7):1032–7.
152. Levine WN, Djurasovic M, Glasson JM, Pollock RG, Flatow EL, Bigliani LU. Hemiarthroplasty for glenohumeral osteoarthritis: results correlated to degree of glenoid wear. J Shoulder Elbow Surg. 1997;6:449–54.
153. Hettrich CM, Weldon E III, Boorman RS, Parsons IM IV, Matsen FA III. Preoperative factors associated with improvements in shoulder function after humeral hemiarthroplasty. J Bone Joint Surg Am. 2004;86:1446–51.
154. Denard PJ, Wirth MA, Orfaly RM. Management of glenohumeral arthritis in the young adult. J Bone Joint Surg Am. 2011;93(9):885–92.
155. Chillemi C, Franceschini V. Shoulder osteoarthritis. Arthritis. 2013;2013:370231.
156. LP MC III, Cole BJ. Nonarthroplasty treatment of glenohumeral cartilage lesions. Arthroscopy. 2005;21(9):1131–42.
157. Izquierdo R, Voloshin I, Edwards S, Freehill MQ, Stanwood W, Wiater JM, Watters WC III, Goldberg MJ, Keith M, Turkelson CM, Wies JL, Anderson S, Boyer K, Raymond L, Sluka P, American Academy of Orthopedic Surgeons. Treatment of glenohumeral osteoarthritis. J Am Acad Orthop Surg. 2010;18(6):375–82.
158. Namdari S, Skelley N, Keener JD, Galatz LM, Yamaguchi K. What is the role of arthroscopic debridement for glenohumeral arthritis? A critical examination of the literature. Arthroscopy. 2013;29(8):1392–8.

159. Skelley NW, Namdari S, Chamberlain AM, Keener JD, Galatz LM, Yamaguchi K. Arthroscopic debridement and capsular release for the treatment of shoulder osteoarthritis. Arthroscopy. 2015;31:494–500.
160. Van der Meijden OA, Gaskill TR, Millett PJ. Glenohumeral joint preservation: a review of management options for young, active patients with osteoarthritis. Adv Orthop. 2012;2012:160923. (9 pages)
161. Savoie FH III, Brislin KJ, Argo D. Arthroscopic glenoid resurfacing as a surgical treatment for glenohumeral arthritis in the young patient: midterm results. Arthroscopy. 2009;25(8):864–71.
162. Strauss EJ, Verma NN, Salata MJ, McGill KC, Klifto C, Nicholson GP, Cole BJ, Romeo AA. The high failure rate of biologic resurfacing of the glenoid in young patients with glenohumeral arthritis. J Shoulder Elbow Surg. 2014;23(3):409–19.
163. Lee BK, Vaishnav S, Rick Hatch GF III, Itamura JM. Biologic resurfacing of the glenoid with meniscal allograft: long-term results with minimum 2-year follow-up. J Shoulder Elbow Surg. 2013;22(2):253–60.
164. Elhassan B, Ozbaydar M, Diller D, Higgins LD, Warner JJ. Soft-tissue resurfacing of the glenoid in the treatment of glenohumeral arthritis in active patients less than fifty years old. J Bone Joint Surg Am. 2009;91(2):419–24.
165. Gross CE, Chalmers PN, Chahal J, Van Thiel G, Bach BR Jr, Cole BJ, Romeo AA. Operative treatment of chondral defects in the glenohumeral joint. Arthroscopy. 2012;28(12):1889–901.
166. Bryant D, Litchfield R, Sandow M, Gartsman GM, Guyatt G, Kirkley A. A comparison of pain, strength, range of motion, and functional outcomes after hemiarthroplasty and total shoulder arthroplasty in patients with osteoarthritis of the shoulder. A systematic review and meta-analysis. J Bone Joint Surg Am. 2005;87(9):1947–56.
167. Iannotti JP, Norris TR. Influence of preoperative factors on outcome of shoulder arthroplasty for glenohumeral osteoarthritis. J Bone Joint Surg Am. 2003;85:251–8.
168. McCarty EC, Marx RG, Maerz D, Altchek D, Warren RF. Sports participation after shoulder replacement surgery. Am J Sports Med. 2008;36:1577–81.
169. Bülhoff M, Sattler P, Bruckner T, Loew M, Zeifang F, Raiss P. Do patients return to sports and work after total shoulder replacement surgery? Am J Sports Med. 2015;43:423–7.
170. Papaliodis D, Richardson N, Tartaglione J, Roberts T, Whipple R, Zanaros G. Impact of total shoulder arthroplasty on golfing activity. Clin J Sport Med. 2015;25:338–40.

Chapter 11
The Management of Distal Radius Fractures in the Aging Athlete

Brent Schultz and Robert J. Goitz

Introduction

Distal radius fractures (DRF) in the elderly are common (over 85,000 beneficiaries from Medicare sustain DRF each year [1–3]. As life expectancy increases and people over 65 maintain more active lifestyles, the importance of optimal management of distal radius fractures in the aging population is a question germane not only to the sports doctor but society in general [1, 4].

Over the past 10 years, there was a trend toward internal fixation for the treatment of most unstable distal radius fractures due to the emergence of locked plates which provide a stable reduction, alleviate the need for casting, and allow for a faster return to activities [4–7]. However, there is a higher rate of complications and less data available for the elderly [4, 7–10].

In the face of multiple treatment options, this chapter will address two questions: (1) how does one best treat fractures of the distal radius in the aging population, and (2) does athletic status potentially alter these treatment pathways?

Scientific Evidence

To address the first question, evidence supports that radiographic alignment of the healed distal radius directly correlates with outcomes in populations younger than 65 years of age [4, 11–13]. Furthermore, better radiographic alignment is more consistently achieved with plate fixation in distal radius fractures [6, 8, 12–14].

B. Schultz, MD · R. J. Goitz, MD (✉)
Department of Orthopaedic Surgery, University of Pittsburgh Medical Center (UPMC), Pittsburgh, PA, USA
e-mail: goitzrj@upmc.edu

© Springer International Publishing AG, part of Springer Nature 2018
V. J. Wright, K. K. Middleton (eds.), *Masterful Care of the Aging Athlete*,
https://doi.org/10.1007/978-3-319-16223-2_11

135

Surgeons have extrapolated this data to the treatment of the elderly [15, 16], which has led to an increase in the treatment of DRF with operative intervention. In 1997, 83% of DRF in the Medicare population were treated in a closed fashion and 1% with internal fixation. By 2005, closed treatment decreased to 70%, and the use of internal fixation rose to 16% [1].

However, practice trends do not necessarily correlate with scientific evidence in the elderly. It must be noted that a number of small studies outlined above do not support the idea that data derived from younger populations can be directly applied to individuals over the age of 65 [17] and that cast management and operative intervention may be equivalent in the older populations [4, 8–10]. In fact, the non-superiority of operative treatment in the elderly population compared to closed management of unstable distal radius fractures is central to the management controversy.

There is evidence suggesting that even unstable DRF should be managed non-operatively in the elderly because anatomic alignment by radiographs does not correlate with functional outcomes. Furthermore, there was no level 1 evidence studying the question of DRF in the elderly until 2011 [4]. Given that this study potentially offers the best evidence regarding DRF in the elderly, we will summarize their results here.

Seventy-one patients over the age of 65 with unstable distal radius fractures were prospectively randomized to surgery or a cast. Surgery did not clearly demonstrate a long-term benefit. Lower DASH scores in the operative group were noted in the early postoperative period, but no differences were detected at 6- and 12-month follow-up. Radiographic parameters were superior in the operative group $p < .05$ at all-time points. However, complications were higher in the operative group of 13 compared to 5 out of 73 patients. Posttreatment osteoarthritis was higher in all non-op groups regardless of the articular involvement of the fracture. However, no differences in self-reported pain levels were found.

Regarding complications, no plate failures or non-unions were noted. Five patients experienced extensor tenosynovitis from prominent locking screws. Four patients developed flexor tenosynovitis from the volar plate placed distal to the watershed region. One EPL tendon rupture from screw penetration was reported. Complex regional pain syndrome (CRPS) was noted in two operative and five non-operative patients [4]. The only consistent advantage noted in the operative group was a higher grip strength that was higher at all-time points. Improved grip strength in the operative group for unstable DRF in the elderly was echoed elsewhere in the literature [1, 4, 7].

Furthermore, Lutz et al. [9] suggested in a 2014 study of 129 matched patients for fracture severity, age, and sex that there was a higher complication rate in the operative group than in the non-operative group, with no statistical benefit measured by the DASH or the PRWE. This data further places operative management into question for patients over 65 with unstable DRF.

What was generally agreed upon is that stable fractures in the elderly can be treated with cast immobilization alone [4, 8, 10, 17]. Furthermore, the evidence suggests that in the elderly, closed treatment of stable fractures leads to equivalent outcomes to ORIF of unstable fractures [10].

Bone Density

Elderly women are typically most at risk for fragility fractures of the distal radius; however, the average DRF patient in the retired population is a 66-year-old female with diminished bone density [1, 2]. The average person represented in Medicare data [1, 2], or the studies cited thus far, may not accurately represent the physiology of an athlete who also happens to be over the age of 65. In fact, data generated from over 600 senior Olympic athletes in Pittsburgh found that 59% of the oldest (>80-year-old) female athletes maintained normal bone density [18]. Therefore, senior athletes by virtue of their increased activity were able to maintain their bone density [18, 19].

This bone density data suggests that aging athletes likely have more youthful bone physiology and potentially have higher demands from their hands as manifest in higher bone densities. These possibilities also suggest that the optimal reduction and fixation of a DRF in an aging athlete may be of greater value than in his or her nonathletic counterpart.

Factors to Consider in Counseling the Aging Athlete

When counseling a senior athlete having sustained a DRF, it is important to inform them that their recovery will be extended compared to younger individuals: patients younger than 65 required 6 months to reach maximal recovery following volar locking plate, while the elderly continued to recover for 12 months [7]. However, the prolonged recovery of elderly patients in general, following DRF, may also justify ORIF in the elderly athlete. As recovery times are perhaps doubled compared to younger patients, an emphasis on early rehabilitation may optimize the aging athletes overall outcome.

Arora et al. [4] demonstrated, in the only randomized controlled trial of operative versus non-operative treatment of unstable DRFs in the elderly, that the DASH and PRWE scores were lower in the operative group at 6 and 12 weeks ($p = .05$), although the DASH scores were equivalent at 3 and 6 months when comparing operative to non-operative groups. A faster early recovery could be an advantage in elderly athletes.

These senior individuals may benefit from a faster recovery to get back to their sport, maintain their higher level of bone density, and maintain better overall mental and physical well-being. Furthermore, we believe that hand dominance as well as the nature of the sport should also factor into the decision-making process to proceed to surgery. If a patient injured the dominant hand in a sport that is upper extremity intensive, such as racquet sports, golf, weight lifting, etc., the early return to motion and strengthening afforded by rigid fixation is a compelling benefit.

Surgical Considerations

Presuming that an aging athlete is deemed an appropriate candidate for surgery following DRF, indications and treatment goals focus on anatomic reduction of the fracture, stable fixation, and early range of motion [5, 6, 13, 14, 20]. The strongest predictor of functional outcome is the quality of the reduction [13]. Furthermore, failure to obtain these parameters following closed reduction is the primary indication for operative management [5, 6, 13, 14, 20].

Intra-articular step offs and gaps of the distal radius are both significant predictors of functional outcome, specifically long-term range of motion [13, 21]. Regarding extra articular components of fractures, radial shortening correlates strongly with long-term grip strength [11, 13, 20, 22–24]. Palmar tilt is associated with higher overall DASH scores, but ulnar variance is one of the strongest predictors of diminished functional capacity [11, 13, 20, 22–24]. Associated ulnar styloid fractures do not generally affect postoperative outcomes, but overall severity of the preoperative distal radius fracture does correlate with long-term results [13]. Associated scapho-lunate ligament injuries in the elderly are generally ignored since their long-term outcome, resulting in SLAC wrist arthritis, generally takes upward of 5–10 years to develop, and its operative treatment would prolong recovery with uncertain short-term benefits.

Surgical Indications

Below is a summary of the most commonly cited indications for operative reduction [6]. Furthermore, the goal of surgery is to eliminate any of the below abnormalities on postoperative radiographs:

- Ulnar variance >1–2 mm positive
- Dorsal tilt >10°–15°
- Radial inclination <10°–15°
- Significant comminution or malalignment of articular surface (>2 mm displaced gap or step off)
- Associated scaphoid fracture
- Any fracture treated closed that loses reduction and now satisfies any of the above criteria

Surgical Fixation Options

There are multiple operative approaches available for the treatment of DRF. These range from closed reduction with percutaneous pinning and cast immobilization to pinning with external fixation to internal plate fixation. The current trend leans strongly toward volar-locked plating systems as these techniques allow for rigid anatomic reduction and early range of motion [6, 7, 15, 16, 23].

Standard Surgical Approach

The standard approach is through the flexor carpi radialis (FCR) sub-sheath. First, an incision is made designed over the FCR from the distal wrist crease coursing proximally for approximately 5–6 cm. The FCR tendon sheath is incised along the entire course of the incision, thus retracting the tendon ulnarly. The floor of the FCR sheath is then incised. The finger flexor tendons and median nerve are retracted ulnarly, and the radial artery is retracted radially. A combination of sharp and blunt dissection is then utilized to identify and ulnarly retract the pronator quadratus (PQ) and flexor pollicis longus (PL). Often, elements of the PQ are interposed in the fracture and must be removed to effect an anatomic reduction. If one finds it difficult to obtain proper reduction of the radial styloid fragment, and thus, achieve full radial height, a brachioradialis (BR) tenotomy may be considered. BR tenotomies have not been shown to affect elbow flexion strength in long-term follow-up of DRF patients undergoing ORIF [25]. Once the fracture is fully debrided of soft tissue, reduction is obtained using a combination of longitudinal traction and direct fracture fragment manipulation. This may be aided with the use of a bone clamp on the proximal radius fragment, which will aid in pronating the distal fragments. Volar plating is performed according to the manufacturer's specifications. Emphasis must be placed on anatomic reduction, rigid fixation of the styloid fragment, as well as stabilization of the volar and potentially dorsal ulnar corner fragments. An evaluation of the DRUJ must be performed following fixation of the distal radius and, if found to be unstable, should be addressed.

To avoid the late complications of extensor tendon ruptures, the EPL being at highest risk, all volar distal screws should be unicortical, and care should be taken to not drill beyond the dorsal cortex. Furthermore, the distal lip of the volar plate should not extend beyond the watershed line as flexor tendon irritations and ruptures were reported [26, 27]. Those tendons at greatest risk of rupture from volar hardware placed beyond the watershed line are the flexor digitorum profundus (FDP) and FPL.

Rehabilitation

Immediately postoperative, the patient is instructed to initiate digital, active, and passive range of motion (A/PROM) exercises. If the surgeon is confident of fixation rigidity at 2 weeks, the patient should be transitioned to a removable volar wrist splint and start wrist A/PROM exercises. With clinical evidence of healing, strengthening exercises can be initiated at 6 weeks postoperatively with discontinuation of the splint.

Non-operative, cast treatment generally requires 6 weeks of immobilization. Next, a removable splint is employed for 2 weeks with the initiation of aggressive A/PROM exercises. Strengthening and more aggressive ROM usually begin at 8 weeks post-injury.

Case Scenario

A 72-year-old right-handed man sustained a three-part right intra-articular DRF with dorsal comminution, 20° dorsal tilt, and a 2 mm gap between the scaphoid and lunate facets with 2 mm ulna positive variance after falling from his bicycle. He takes lisinopril for hypertensive control and a prophylactic baby aspirin. No other major medical comorbidities are noted. He is a retired business executive, competitive squash player, and bicycling enthusiast. What is the most reasonable option for this patient?

His ulna positive variance makes him most at risk for long-term ulna wrist pain, and the articular displacement with significant dorsal tilt will result in diminished grip strength. The literature does not clearly support operative intervention of DRF in patients over 65; however, this healthy athletic individual may not strongly resemble the population from which the studies were performed. Given a lack of information on athletic seniors regarding DRF, the key to optimizing the management of this patient is to fully inform him of his potential options.

Closed cast management is justified in the literature, but the patient will likely sustain a loss of grip strength (4 lbs on average) without ORIF and will have greater disability in the early phase of treatment of up to 3 months. Also, early active range of motion will be precluded. The patient should also be informed that any residual deformity after a closed reduction will not correct itself with cast management alone.

Given the significant articular involvement, unstable nature of the fracture, high-demand lifestyle, and dominant hand involvement, we believe that offering this patient an open reduction with volar locking plate is entirely reasonable to optimize his return to his pre-injury functional level. Before making this decision, the patient should be informed that an operation may place him at higher risk for hardware-related complications (potentially even requiring reoperation) for a benefit that was not studied in his specific patient population but rather extrapolated from a younger cohort.

References

1. Shauver MJ, Yin H, Banerjee M, Chung KC. Current and future national costs to medicare for the treatment of distal radius fracture in the elderly. J Hand Surg Am. 2011;36:1282–7.
2. Apex CoVantage LLC. Postmenopausal. 2008;1–4.

3. Shauver MJ, Clapham PJ, Chung KC. An economic analysis of outcomes and complications of treating distal radius fractures in the elderly. J Hand Surg Am. 2011;36:1912–8.e3.
4. Arora R, et al. A prospective randomized trial comparing nonoperative treatment with volar locking plate fixation for displaced and unstable distal radial fractures in patients sixty-five years of age and older. J Bone Joint Surg Am. 2011;93(23):2146–53.
5. Grewal R, MacDermid JC, King GJW, Faber KJ. Open reduction internal fixation versus percutaneous pinning with external fixation of distal radius fractures: a prospective, randomized clinical trial. J Hand Surg Am. 2011;36:1899–906.
6. Cherubino P, Bini A, Marcolli D. Management of distal radius fractures: treatment protocol and functional results. Injury. 2010;41:1120–6.
7. Chung KC, Squitieri L, Kim HM. Comparative outcomes study using the volar locking plating system for distal radius fractures in both young adults and adults older than 60 years. J Hand Surg Am. 2008;33:809–19.
8. Arora R, et al. A comparative study of clinical and radiologic outcomes of unstable colles type distal radius fractures in patients older than 70 years: nonoperative treatment versus volar locking plating. J Orthop Trauma. 2009;23:237–42.
9. Lutz K, Yeoh KM, MacDermid JC, Symonette C, Grewal R. Complications associated with operative versus nonsurgical treatment of distal radius fractures in patients aged 65 years and older. J Hand Surg Am. 2014;39:1280–6.
10. Egol KA. Distal radial fractures in the elderly: operative compared with nonoperative treatment. J Bone Joint Surg Am. 2010;92:1851.
11. McQueen M, Caspers J. Colles fracture: does the anatomical result affect the final function? J Bone Joint Surg Br. 1988;70:649–51.
12. Rozental TD, et al. Functional outcomes for unstable distal radial fractures treated with open reduction and internal fixation or closed reduction and percutaneous fixation: a prospective randomized trial. J Bone Joint Surg Am. 2009;91:1837–46.
13. Trumble TE, Schmitt SR, Vedder NB. Factors affecting functional outcome of displaced intra-articular distal radius fractures. J Hand Surg Am. 1994;19:325–40.
14. Kreder HJ, et al. A randomized, controlled trial of distal radius fractures with metaphyseal displacement but without joint incongruity: closed reduction and casting versus closed reduction, spanning external fixation, and optional percutaneous K-wires. J Orthop Trauma. 2006;20:115–21.
15. Orbay JL, Fernandez DL. Volar fixation for dorsally displaced fractures of the distal radius: a preliminary report. J Hand Surg Am. 2002;27:205–15.
16. Orbay JL, Fernandez DL. Volar fixed-angle plate fixation for unstable distal radius fractures in the elderly patient. J Hand Surg Am. 2004;29:96–102.
17. Grewal R, MacDermid JC. The risk of adverse outcomes in extra-articular distal radius fractures is increased with malalignment in patients of all ages but mitigated in older patients. J Hand Surg Am. 2007;32:962–70.
18. Leigey D, Irrgang J, Francis K, Cohen P, Wright V. Participation in high-impact sports predicts bone mineral density in Senior Olympic Athletes. Sports Health: A Multidisciplinary Approach. 2009;1:508–13.
19. Velez NF, et al. The effect of moderate impact exercise on skeletal integrity in master athletes. Osteoporos Int. 2008;19:1457–64.
20. Batra S, Gupta A. The effect of fracture-related factors on the functional outcome at 1 year in distal radius fractures. Injury. 2002;33:499–502.
21. Knirk JL, Jupiter JBA. Intra-articular fractures of the distal end of the radius in young adults. J Bone Joint Surg Am. 1986;68:647–59.
22. McQueen MM, Hajducka C, Court-Brown CM. Redisplaced unstable fractures of the distal radius: a prospective randomised comparison of four methods of treatment. J Bone Joint Surg Br. 1996;78:404–9.
23. Keating JF, Court-Brown CM, McQueen MM. Internal fixation of volar-displaced distal radial fractures. J Bone Joint Surg Br. 1994;76:401–5.

24. van der Linden W, Ericson RA. Colles' fracture. How should its displacement be measured and how should it be immobilized? J Bone Joint Surg Am. 1981;63:1285–8.
25. Kim JK, Park JS, Shin SJ, Bae H, Kim SY. The effect of brachioradialis release during distal radius fracture fixation on elbow flexion strength and wrist function. J Hand Surg Am. 2014;39(11):2246–50.
26. Soong M. Volar locking plate implant prominence and flexor tendon rupture. J Bone Joint Surg Am. 2011;93:328.
27. Asadollahi S, Keith PPA. Flexor tendon injuries following plate fixation of distal radius fractures: a systematic review of the literature. J Orthop Traumatol. 2013;14:227–34.

Chapter 12
Foot and Ankle: Conservative Management, Operative Management, and Return to Sport

Monique C. Chambers, Dukens LaBaze, Jesse Raszeswki, and MaCalus V. Hogan

Achilles Tendon Injury

Introduction

Achilles tendinopathy is one of the most frequent foot and ankle injuries that results from overuse [1]. Achilles tendon ruptures occur more commonly in healthy, active individuals with a mean age of 37 years [2]. Achilles injury is more likely present in running and jumping activities, with rates as high as 9% in recreational runners [1]. It has an incidence of 5.6% in nonathletes [1]. Males are predisposed with as high as a 30:1 ratio to women [2]. Achilles tendinopathy can occur at two anatomical locations: *insertional* tendinopathy at the calcaneus-Achilles tendon junction or *non-insertional* tendinopathy which is approximately 2–6 cm proximal to the insertion site of the Achilles tendon [1]. Insertional tendinopathy tends to occur in active individuals, whereas non-insertional is more frequently observed in older, less active, and overweight individuals [1].

Tendinous fibers from the gastrocnemius and the soleus muscles coalesce toward the calcaneal tuberosity to form the Achilles tendon, which is the largest tendon in the body [3]. The tendon spans three separate joints and is integral for knee flexion,

M. C. Chambers, MD, MSL · D. LaBaze, BS
Department of Orthopaedic Surgery, University of Pittsburgh Medical Center, Pittsburgh, PA, USA

J. Raszeswki, MBS
Alabama College of Osteopathic Medicine, Dothan, AL, USA
e-mail: raszewskija@acomedu.org

M. V. Hogan, MD (✉)
Foot and Ankle Division, Department of Orthopedic Surgery, University of Pittsburgh Medical Center, Pittsburgh, PA, USA
e-mail: hoganmv@upmc.edu

© Springer International Publishing AG, part of Springer Nature 2018
V. J. Wright, K. K. Middleton (eds.), *Masterful Care of the Aging Athlete*,
https://doi.org/10.1007/978-3-319-16223-2_12

foot plantar flexion, and hind foot inversion [2]. The normal blood supply is variable but is derived from three sources: the muscle-tendon junction, the bone-tendon junction, and the length of the tendon [1]. The most important blood supply derives from the paratenon in the middle zone, with the most abundant blood supply located at the insertion [1]. This distribution of the blood supply leaves the Achilles tendon prone to injury in the watershed area approximately 2–6 cm from its insertion on the posterior calcaneus [4]. The tibial nerve supplies the superficial and deep nerves to local tissues that innervate the Achilles tendon [1].

Insertional tendinopathy is due to the degeneration of the tendon at the insertion on the calcaneus, stemming from old age, steroid use, obesity, diabetes, and inflammatory arthropathies [2]. Conservative treatment, activity modification, is the mainstay of therapy. When surgical intervention is necessary, a posterior central tendon approach for debridement of the tendon with removal of the prominent calcaneal projection is often utilized [2].

Non-insertional Achilles tendinopathy is due to an inflammatory reaction that leads to circulatory impairment and edema, which can progress to fibrinous adhesions in the chronic state [2]. Conservative management is also the mainstay of therapy, with activity modifications, eccentric exercises, NSAIDs, injections, and shock wave therapy [2]. If pain is not alleviated with conservative measures, surgical intervention can be used. Surgical treatment includes debridement and excision of the fibrous adhesions, with the goal of denervating and devascularizing the paratenon while promoting a scarring response within the tendon [2].

Achilles tendinopathy is often multifactorial in origin, and the risk factors can be divided into intrinsic and extrinsic factors. Intrinsic factors include biomechanical abnormalities of the lower extremity, and extrinsic factors include excessive mechanical overload and training errors [1]. For intrinsic examples, individuals with hyper-pronation or cavus feet are prone to higher incidence of Achilles tendon problems [3]. Advanced age also correlates with Achilles tendinopathy. As for extrinsic factors, individuals that use footwear with insufficient heel height or inadequate shock absorption have been shown to magnify the stress placed on the Achilles tendon during athletic activity [3]. Achilles tendinopathy is severely debilitating, and injuries can have a substantial socioeconomic impact regardless of the treatment selected [4].

In this chapter, the clinical presentation, physical examination, diagnostic work-up, and treatments will be reviewed and illustrated (Table 12.1).

Table 12.1 Features of Achilles tendinopathy

Clinical manifestations	• Pain in the posterior aspect of the foot/ankle • Pain with plantar flexion motion • Inability to bear weight
Diagnosis	• Inability to perform single-leg raise • Confirm with MRI/ultrasound
Treatment	• Tendinopathy → physical therapy • Anatomical deformity (tear/rupture) → surgery

Clinical Evaluation

Achilles tendinopathy is primarily diagnosed based on history and physical exam. Patients usually describe sudden onset of pain in the posterior aspect of the foot and ankle, with activities that incorporate forceful plantar flexion [4]. Patients who have ruptured the tendon often have a "pop" sensation, lose the ability to bear weight, and report sudden weakness in plantar flexion of the ankle [4]. Sufficient evaluation of the Achilles tendon requires bilateral examination of the foot and ankle while the patient is standing, ambulating, and prone with their feet suspended over the edge of an examination table.

A complete musculoskeletal examination entails thorough inspection and palpation of both feet and ankles with side-by-side comparisons for reference. Begin by inspecting the posterior ankle for signs of fracture, sprain, or tendon rupture, which are typically associated with bruising, swelling, and/or foot misalignment. Also, assess for peripheral artery disease, which presents as dry, shiny, hairless, hyperpigmented, or edematous skin. Evaluate for signs of poor gait mechanics, evidenced by asymmetric diminution of the patient's footwear, foot deformity, and leg-length discrepancy [5].

Next, palpate the Achilles tendon in plantar flexion, dorsiflexion, and neutral position. Engage the proximal aspect between the thumb and index finger, applying mild pressure in a stepwise fashion distally toward the insertion site on the calcaneus. Assess for tenderness, defects, thickening, and crepitus, remaining aware that the presence of edema or hematoma may result in false-negative examination.

Examination should be conducted with the patient prone and the feet hanging off the ledge of the examination table [3]. The entire gastrocnemius-soleus-myotendinous complex should be thoroughly palpated, while the ankle is gently maneuvered through active and passive ranges of motion [3]. Positive physical examination findings include increased passive ankle dorsiflexion, weak plantar flexion strength, and palpable defect overlying a tear [4].

Location can help differentiate tendinopathy from other causes of posterior ankle tenderness. Tendinopathy classically exhibits a pattern of localized tenderness 2–6 cm proximally from the calcaneal insertion site as well as crepitus with motion. Tenderness directly on the Achilles tendon at the insertion site is more consistent with enthesopathy. Tenderness and warmth at the insertion site, superficial to the Achilles tendon, is more consistent with subcutaneous calcaneal bursitis. Tenderness and warmth at the insertion site, deep to the Achilles tendon, is more consistent with subtendinous bursitis (retrocalcaneal bursitis), which can be evaluated by grasping and laterally displacing the Achilles tendon with one hand while palpating the underlying soft tissue with the contralateral hand [6]. The American Academy of Orthopaedic Surgeons (AAOS) clinical practice guidelines note that a diagnosis can be made when two or more of the following exam findings are noted: a positive Thompson test (when compression of the calf in supine position does not elicit passive plantar flexion), decreased plantar flexion strength, palpable defect distal to insertion site, or positive Matles test (increased passive ankle dorsiflexion at rest) [2].

Potential for misdiagnosis of tendon pathology on physical examination exists in the presence of certain signs and symptoms: intact active plantar flexion of the foot, intact ambulation, absence of pain, and undetectable Achilles tendon defects on examination. In fact, 20–30% of ruptured Achilles tendons are missed during evaluation due to the patients' ability to ambulate and actively plantar flex the ankle [7].

Imaging studies, such as MRI and ultrasound, can be utilized to confirm physical exam findings. MRI is one of the most useful imaging tools because it allows for evaluation of the Achilles tendon in the sagittal plane to determine the length of the injured or diseased tendon and subsequent surgical planning. MRI has a sensitivity of 95% and a specificity of 50% when evaluating Achilles tendon pathology [8]. Ultrasound can verify the existence and location of intra-tendinous lesions. Ultrasound provides many advantages, quick, safe, and inexpensive, but also has many disadvantages being operator-dependent and not as readily accessible. Plain radiographs can also be used to evaluate retrocalcaneal bursitis and a possible Haglund's deformity, which is a prominence of the posterosuperior angle of the os calcis that causes mechanical irritation of the retrocalcaneal bursa that can exacerbate Achilles tendinopathy [8].

Nonoperative Treatment

The purpose of conservative treatment is to facilitate the return to activity and manage symptoms. Nonsteroidal anti-inflammatory drugs (NSAIDs) can be a good short-term option for pain management. Steroid injections have also been used to provide some short-term relief; however, Achilles tendon rupture has been observed following these injections and are usually avoided [9].

A number of studies have demonstrated significantly improved outcomes with the use of eccentric exercise training. Eccentric heel-drop training (ECC) for 6 weeks exhibited a patient satisfaction score of >7 in more than 80% of patients, return to premorbid activity on average of 10 weeks. Additionally pain scores as measured by visual analog score (VAS) decreased from 7.2 at initiation to 2.9 after 6 weeks and 1.1 after 6 months [10]. Eccentric exercise for 12 weeks as the sole treatment for Achilles tendinopathy demonstrated clear changes to objective assessments of inflammation on MRI, tendon volume decreases from 6.6 ± 3.1 cm^3 to 5.8 ± 2.3 cm on T1-weighted images, and proton density on average decreased 23% [11]. Another study assessed changes to the Achilles tendon after 12 weeks of eccentric exercise using ultrasonography (US). At the widest portion of the Achilles tendon, patients in the ECC group showed significant changes compared to the control group, with change from 8.8 to 7.6 mm. Additionally, after exercise treatment 73% of the ECC subjects had normal Achilles tendon anatomy on US after treatment compared to the hypoechoic areas present at onset of the study [12].

Heavy slow resistance (HSR) training is another exercise treatment option. In a randomized control trial, comparing HSR to ECC, both groups showed improvement on US, the Victorian Institute of Sport Assessment-Achilles (VISA-A) questionnaire, and VAS scores. Patients in the HSR group were more satisfied at 12 weeks and were significantly more compliant. Differences in satisfaction and compliance may be attributed to the time commitments for each. HSR required three 36-min training sessions per week, whereas ECC required two 22-min training sessions per day, 7 days a week [13].

Shoe modifications are commonly recommended to reduce Achilles tendon strain, promote movement variability of the hind foot, and correct eversion of the calcaneus when there is excessive pronation. Munteanu et al. conducted a randomized control trial comparing customized foot orthoses to sham orthoses and found no difference in the mean VISA-A score between groups, 82.1 ± 16.3 and 79.2 ± 20.0, respectively [14]. Night splints are also an effective treatment option, but are not as effective in return to play at 12 weeks and pain reduction when compared to ECC. There is no additive effect observed when night splints are used in conjunction with ECC [15].

Low-level laser therapy (LLLT) has demonstrated anti-inflammatory, regenerative, and anti-apoptotic properties. The use of LLLT in conjunction with ECC accelerates recovery faster than ECC alone. Extracorporeal shock wave therapy (ESWT) is another promising treatment option that improves VISA-A, VAS, and Likert scores; ESWT also has an additive effect when combined with ECC. Platelet-rich plasma (PRP) is a highly researched topic garnering much attention. PRP is beneficial to other tendinopathies. However, currently there are no RCTs that show significant improvement with the use of PRP specifically for Achilles tendon injuries [16].

Operative Treatment

Once patients fail conservative management, appropriate indications for surgical repair are evaluated. Operative treatment is pursued based on the nature and acuity of the injury. For patients that have sustained an acute rupture, undergo surgical repair once the initial swelling and ecchymosis subsides. In a meta-analysis performed by Bhandari et al., surgical repair showed a significant reduction in the risk of re-rupture compared to conservative treatment [17]. However, surgical repair increases the rate of infection. There were no major differences in return to normal function following rehabilitation.

For patients with chronic Achilles tendinopathy, there is much controversy regarding the approach (tendoscopy vs. open), the type of suture method, and need for augmentation. Percutaneous repair has shown to have lower infection rates than open repair, and the re-rupture rate of 2% is lower [18]. However, there is also an increased risk of damage or injury to the sural nerve. Re-rupture risk is partially related to the gap distance between the ends of the tendon and early weight bearing in the postoperative period [19].

Although simple end-to-end repair is common, evidence to support the use of augmentation has been increasing in the literature. Nonetheless, superiority of augmented tendon repair has yet to be established. A recent meta-analysis showed no major difference in outcomes of patients with augmented versus repairs without augmentation. Patients had no statistically significant difference for re-rupture rates, patient satisfaction, return to activity, or infection rate [20].

Conclusion

Injuries to the Achilles tendon can be debilitating for the masters athletes. Thorough assessment of the extent of damage to the structure is required. Appropriate patient selection for surgical intervention is necessary to achieve the best possible outcomes for athletic performance and to minimize unnecessary risk of infection associated with more of an aggressive approach. Most athletes can expect to return to sport around 6 months postoperatively and regain full function between 9 and 12 months after surgery.

Plantar Fasciitis

Introduction

Plantar fasciitis is a common condition leading to more than one million clinical visits per year. Approximately 60% of those visits were patients 45 years of age or older with patients between the ages of 45 and 64 having two times the average incidence of 8.2 per 1000 persons [21]. The reported prevalence of plantar fasciitis in runners is as high as 10% [22].

Clinical Evaluation

Patients with plantar fasciitis often complain of an insidious onset of pain on the plantar surface of the heel. The pain is worse with the first step down after sleeping and improves as they walk and my worsen at the end of the day. On exam, they may be observed walking on their toes, as this relieves the aching and tearing type of pressure from the fascia. Tenderness to palpation occurs at the plantar fascia insertion site on the medial tuberosity of the calcaneus, particularly with dorsiflexion of the forefoot. A tight Achilles tendon may also be noted on exam.

Nonoperative Treatment

First-line treatment is plantar fascia stretching and Achilles tendon stretching. Patients on a plantar fascia stretching protocol have VAS scores that reflect significantly reduced pain when compared to Achilles tendon stretching alone, although this effect is not sustained at 2-year follow-up [23]. The plantar stretch is performed by having the patient position their fingers at the base of the toes, with the toes dorsiflexed while using a free hand to apply tension on the toes until a stretch is felt in the arch. Patients are encouraged to stretch before taking their first steps in the morning and after extended period of weight bearing that leads to pain [23, 24]. A tennis ball can also be used to assist with stretching and pressure massage of the scar tissue. NSAIDs can be added to the treatment regimen, but there is currently no literature to support the use of NSAIDs as the sole treatment for plantar fasciitis [25]. Cryotherapy application for 20 min at bedtime reduces pain and has been shown to have a significant impact when used in conjunction with NSAIDs [26].

The use of orthoses in the treatment of plantar fasciitis is common and in combination with stretching has better outcomes than stretching alone [27]. A study looking at patients 65 years of age or older demonstrated that prefabricated foot orthosis are the best at reducing pressure on heel and is 5 times better at pressure reduction than heel inserts or heel pad [28].

Injections are another line of treatment available for patients. Corticosteroid injections can provide relief of symptoms for several months. However, corticosteroids increase the risk of plantar fascia rupture and chances compound with more injections [29, 30]. Botulinum toxin A (BTX-A) is a novel injection option that has exhibited the ability to reduce pain and increase function up to 1 year. At 6 months, BTX-A on average decreased VAS scores from 7.2 to 3.6 and increased Foot and Ankle Ability Measure (FAAM) from 36.3 to 73.8 [31]. Though more long-term studies are needed to assess BTX-A injections, it currently has less side-effects than steroids.

Extracorporeal shock wave therapy (ESWT) is an FDA-approved treatment option for plantar fasciitis. A randomized control trial demonstrated significant difference in VAS and Roles and Maudsley scores in middle-aged patients treated with ESWT compared to placebo group, with a success rate of 50–65%. Temporary swelling and pain during treatment were the only device-related unfavorable events observed [32].

Operative Treatment

When all other conservative options are exhausted, then surgery becomes an option. Plantar fasciotomy is a regularly performed procedure for this condition and requires persistent pain after 9 months of failed conservative measures. This procedure has an outcome success rate up to 90% for distal tarsal tunnel decompression and dual plantar fascial release. This procedure may result in prolonged heal healing and rehabilitation time. Plantar fascia release is thought to decrease foot arch and ankle stability [24].

Conclusion

Irritation of the plantar fascia occurs in many athletes. Inflammatory flares results in nagging pain that can prevent continuous activity, especially in runners. Aggressive stretching and therapy are required to minimize the limits on exercise. Injections are usually avoided to minimize the risk of rupture. For patients that undergo fasciotomy with or without tarsal tunnel decompression, success rates are high, 70–80% with a full return to activity expected. However, complications and slower recovery often occur and should be thoroughly considered prior to surgical intervention.

Stress Fractures

Introduction

Stress fractures are a common sports injury that account for 10% of all sports injuries, with as many as 30% of injuries in like runners and ballet dancers. They occur in roughly 20% of elite athletes and 1% among recreational athletes. An overwhelming 90% of stress fractures are in the lower extremities [33, 34]. Stress fractures are either low-risk or high-risk; high-risk fractures have increased rates of nonunion/delayed union and tend to be in areas not well vascularized [33–35]. Low-risk fractures tend to be in areas that are well vascularized and carry a decreased risk of nonunion/delayed union.

There are several factors that predispose athletes to stress fractures. Training pattern is a factor that is particularly important for masters athletes. An abrupt increase in training intensity increases probability of stress fractures. This principle has been observed with military cadets who have significantly higher rates of stress fractures during the first week of boot camp training. This phenomenon is also observed in professional soccer leagues, where a shorter preseason resulted in higher rates of stress fractures during high activity in the season [33].

Bone health is a predisposing factor that should be emphasized, particularly with female athletes. Athletes with irregular menstrual cycles can have a relative risk up to four times higher than their eumenorrheic counterparts [36]. Female naval cadets given daily calcium and vitamin D showed a 20% decrease in stress fractures compared to placebo. A similar study compared daily calcium supplementation to placebo in men and revealed no difference in stress fracture rates. Other predisposing factors include biomechanics, training surface, and footwear [33].

Clinical Evaluation

Navicular stress fractures are a common high-risk stress fracture most frequently seen in basketball players, ballet dancers, and runners [37, 38]. Patients usually complain of pinpoint pain that is worse with activity. The pain will usually have an insidious onset that is relieved with limited motion/activity. Approximately 40% of navicular stress fracture changes are absent on radiographs; CT should be used when patients continue to report pain despite negative radiographs [39]. The outcome is correlated to the severity of the fracture, which is assessed by using the Saxena classification (Table 12.2) [40].

Table 12.2 CT findings and treatment based on Saxena classification

Grade	CT findings	Treatment
Type 1	Involves only the dorsal cortex	• NWBC
Type 2	Dorsal cortex and the body are involved	• NWBC • ORIF once NWBC fails
Type 3	Dorsal and volar involvement	• ORIF or fusion

Nonoperative Treatment

There is no consensus on the treatment of navicular stress fractures due to the lack of randomized controlled trials comparing surgical to conservative treatments [22, 35, 37, 38, 40, 41]. The primary nonoperative treatment is the use of a non-weight-bearing cast (NWBC). NWBC for at least 6 weeks has a success rate of 80% in healing the fracture and return to normal activity. Treatment plans that allow patients to bear weight only have a success rate of 29% with higher rates of nonunion, delayed union, and/or refracture [37]. Bone stimulators are used in some elite athletes to accelerate the bone healing process. Bone stimulators cause no harm and have not proven to be beneficial for navicular fractures. However, this method has demonstrated the ability to accelerate healing in tibia and distal radius fractures [41]. Like bone stimulators, shock wave therapy has demonstrated a benefit in other types of osseous injury but lacks evidence for use in stress fractures due to the paucity of literature [41]. The average time of return to play is 21.7 weeks for nonoperative treatment [37].

Operative Treatment

Surgical intervention is indicated for patients with displaced or complete fractures (Saxena Grade III). Patients who undergo surgical fixation have a return to play time of 16.4 weeks and lower rates of nonunion, delayed union, and refracture when compared to nonoperative management [37]. Complications with open reduction and internal fixation (ORIF) include superficial infection, return to OR for removal of hardware, and nonunion [37]. In elite athletes and patients with high functional demands, surgical intervention is favored [41]. Patients with partial fractures observed on CT will improve with inactivity, but may become symptomatic upon return to sport. Surgical intervention reduces the uncertainty associated with nonoperative treatment, while also providing a faster return to play [41].

Conclusions

Stress fractures result from overuse and become more common with repeated force and load, especially as the arch changes over time. For patients that have relief with inactivity, conservative measures such as bone stimulation and vitamin supplementation with vitamin D and calcium are the mainstay of treatment to promote bone healing. However, the navicular bone of the foot represents an area with low healing potential due to the lack of vascularity in the region. Therefore, some patients will require surgical fixation to return to sport. Surgical management of navicular stress fractures may offer a faster return to sport for high-level athletes. Further randomized control trails are needed to establish if this is true for the management of all navicular stress fractures.

References

1. Li HY, Hua YH. Achilles tendinopathy: current concepts about the basic science and clinical treatments. Biomed Res Int. 2016;2016:6492597.
2. Egger AC, Berkowitz MJ. Achilles tendon injuries. Curr Rev Musculoskelet Med. 2017;10(1):72–80.
3. Saltzman CL, Tearse DS. Achilles tendon injuries. J Am Acad Orthop Surg. 1998;6(5):316–25.
4. Pedowitz D, Kirwan G. Achilles tendon ruptures. Curr Rev Musculoskelet Med. 2013;6(4):285–93.
5. Johnston CA, Taunton JE, Lloyd-Smith DR, McKenzie DC. Preventing running injuries. Practical approach for family doctors. Can Fam Physician. 2003;49:1101–9.
6. Schepsis AA, Jones H, Haas AL. Achilles tendon disorders in athletes. Am J Sports Med. 2002;30(2):287–305.
7. Maffulli N. The clinical diagnosis of subcutaneous tear of the Achilles tendon. A prospective study in 174 patients. Am J Sports Med. 1998;26(2):266–70.
8. Reddy SS, Pedowitz DI, Parekh SG, Omar IM, Wapner KL. Surgical treatment for chronic disease and disorders of the Achilles tendon. J Am Acad Orthop Surg. 2009;17(1):3–14.
9. Kleinman M, Gross AE. Achilles tendon rupture following steroid injection. Report of three cases. J Bone Joint Surg Am. 1983;65(9):1345–7.
10. Verrall G, Schofield S, Brustad T. Chronic Achilles tendinopathy treated with eccentric stretching program. Foot Ankle Int. 2011;32(9):843–9.
11. Shalabi A, Kristoffersen-Wilberg M, Svensson L, Aspelin P, Movin T. Eccentric training of the gastrocnemius-soleus complex in chronic Achilles tendinopathy results in decreased tendon volume and intratendinous signal as evaluated by MRI. Am J Sports Med. 2004;32(5):1286–96.
12. Ohberg L, Lorentzon R, Alfredson H. Eccentric training in patients with chronic Achilles tendinosis: normalised tendon structure and decreased thickness at follow up. Br J Sports Med. 2004;38(1):8–11; discussion 11.
13. Beyer R, Kongsgaard M, Hougs Kjaer B, Ohlenschlaeger T, Kjaer M, Magnusson SP. Heavy slow resistance versus eccentric training as treatment for Achilles tendinopathy: a randomized controlled trial. Am J Sports Med. 2015;43(7):1704–11.
14. Munteanu SE, Scott LA, Bonanno DR, et al. Effectiveness of customised foot orthoses for Achilles tendinopathy: a randomised controlled trial. Br J Sports Med. 2015;49(15):989–94.
15. Roos EM, Engstrom M, Lagerquist A, Soderberg B. Clinical improvement after 6 weeks of eccentric exercise in patients with mid-portion Achilles tendinopathy—a randomized trial with 1-year follow-up. Scand J Med Sci Sports. 2004;14(5):286–95.
16. Filardo G, Di Matteo B, Kon E, Merli G, Marcacci M. Platelet-rich plasma in tendon-related disorders: results and indications. Knee Surg Sports Traumatol Arthrosc. 2016:1–16.
17. Bhandari M, Guyatt GH, Siddiqui F, et al. Treatment of acute Achilles tendon ruptures: a systematic overview and metaanalysis. Clin Orthop Relat Res. 2002;400:190–200.
18. Khan RJ, Carey Smith RL. Surgical interventions for treating acute Achilles tendon ruptures. Cochrane Database Syst Rev. 2010;(9):CD003674.

19. Gulati V, Jaggard M, Al-Nammari SS, et al. Management of Achilles tendon injury: a current concepts systematic review. World J Orthop. 2015;6(4):380–6.
20. Zhang YJ, Zhang C, Wang Q, Lin XJ. Augmented versus nonaugmented repair of acute Achilles tendon rupture: a systematic review and meta-analysis. Am J Sports Med. 2017:363546517702872.
21. Riddle DL, Schappert SM. Volume of ambulatory care visits and patterns of care for patients diagnosed with plantar fasciitis: a national study of medical doctors. Foot Ankle Int. 2004;25(5):303–10.
22. Kindred J, Trubey C, Simons SM. Foot injuries in runners. Curr Sports Med Rep. 2011;10(5):249–54.
23. Digiovanni BF, Nawoczenski DA, Malay DP, et al. Plantar fascia-specific stretching exercise improves outcomes in patients with chronic plantar fasciitis. A prospective clinical trial with two-year follow-up. J Bone Joint Surg Am. 2006;88(8):1775–81.
24. Neufeld SK, Cerrato R. Plantar fasciitis: evaluation and treatment. J Am Acad Orthop Surg. 2008;16(6):338–46.
25. Gill LH, Kiebzak GM. Outcome of nonsurgical treatment for plantar fasciitis. Foot Ankle Int. 1996;17(9):527–32.
26. Knobloch K, Grasemann R, Spies M, Vogt PM. Midportion Achilles tendon microcirculation after intermittent combined cryotherapy and compression compared with cryotherapy alone: a randomized trial. Am J Sports Med. 2008;36(11):2128–38.
27. Pfeffer G, Bacchetti P, Deland J, et al. Comparison of custom and prefabricated orthoses in the initial treatment of proximal plantar fasciitis. Foot Ankle Int. 1999;20(4):214–21.
28. Bonanno DR, Landorf KB, Menz HB. Pressure-relieving properties of various shoe inserts in older people with plantar heel pain. Gait Posture. 2011;33(3):385–9.
29. Acevedo JI, Beskin JL. Complications of plantar fascia rupture associated with corticosteroid injection. Foot Ankle Int. 1998;19(2):91–7.
30. Kim C, Cashdollar MR, Mendicino RW, Catanzariti AR, Fuge L. Incidence of plantar fascia ruptures following corticosteroid injection. Foot Ankle Spec. 2010;3(6):335–7.
31. Ahmad J, Ahmad SH, Jones K. Treatment of plantar fasciitis with botulinum toxin. Foot Ankle Int. 2017;38(1):1–7.
32. Gollwitzer H, Saxena A, DiDomenico LA, et al. Clinically relevant effectiveness of focused extracorporeal shock wave therapy in the treatment of chronic plantar fasciitis: a randomized, controlled multicenter study. J Bone Joint Surg Am. 2015;97(9):701–8.
33. Behrens SB, Deren ME, Matson A, Fadale PD, Monchik KO. Stress fractures of the pelvis and legs in athletes: a review. Sports Health. 2013;5(2):165–74.
34. Robertson GA, Wood AM. Lower limb stress fractures in sport: optimising their management and outcome. World J Orthop. 2017;8(3):242–55.
35. Boden BP, Osbahr DC. High-risk stress fractures: evaluation and treatment. J Am Acad Orthop Surg. 2000;8(6):344–53.
36. Beck BR, Matheson GO, Bergman G, et al. Do capacitively coupled electric fields accelerate tibial stress fracture healing? A randomized controlled trial. Am J Sports Med. 2008;36(3):545–53.
37. Mallee WH, Weel H, van Dijk CN, van Tulder MW, Kerkhoffs GM, Lin CW. Surgical versus conservative treatment for high-risk stress fractures of the lower leg (anterior tibial cortex, navicular and fifth metatarsal base): a systematic review. Br J Sports Med. 2015;49(6):370–6.
38. Mann JA, Pedowitz DI. Evaluation and treatment of navicular stress fractures, including nonunions, revision surgery, and persistent pain after treatment. Foot Ankle Clin. 2009;14(2):187–204.
39. Greaney RB, Gerber FH, Laughlin RL, et al. Distribution and natural history of stress fractures in U.S. Marine recruits. Radiology. 1983;146(2):339–46.
40. Saxena A, Fullem B, Hannaford D. Results of treatment of 22 navicular stress fractures and a new proposed radiographic classification system. J Foot Ankle Surg. 2000;39(2):96–103.
41. Shakked RJ, Walters EE, O'Malley MJ. Tarsal navicular stress fractures. Curr Rev Musculoskelet Med. 2017;10(1):122–30.

Chapter 13
Spine Injuries: Conservative Managment, Operative Management and Return to Sport

Chinedu Nwasike, Paul Hong, and Joon Y. Lee

Introduction

Spine injuries in athletes of any age can be a catastrophic event. The severity of injuries can run from minimal with no neurologic sequelae, to permanent quadriplegia and even death. As athletes age, they become more prone to having disorders and maladies of the spine related to degenerative changes. Aging in the spine is a two-pronged process involving both intervertebral disc degeneration and bone mass reduction. Degeneration can often occur in athletes at an earlier age because of repetitive stresses placed on the spine. This is especially true in athletes that participate in collision sports. In this chapter, we will discuss the considerations of spinal maladies in the aging athlete.

Back Pain

Back pain is one of the leading reasons for patients to be held from activity [1]. The lifetime prevalence of back pain is reported to be as high as 85% [2]. Interestingly, back pain is related to both a lack of physical activity and strenuous activity. Studies show that there is a happy medium of physical activity that will minimize back pain [3, 4]. Other risk factors for back pain in the athlete include female sex and increased

C. Nwasike, MD · J. Y. Lee, MD (✉)
Department of Orthopedic Surgery, University of Pittsburgh Medical Center,
Pittsburgh, PA, USA
e-mail: nwasikeco2@upmc.edu; leejy3@upmc.edu

P. Hong, MD
Sutter Medical Group Neurosciences, Sacramento, CA, USA
e-mail: Hongps2@upmc.edu

© Springer International Publishing AG, part of Springer Nature 2018   155
V. J. Wright, K. K. Middleton (eds.), *Masterful Care of the Aging Athlete*,
https://doi.org/10.1007/978-3-319-16223-2_13

age. For many, back pain is a transient event that resolves with no treatment; however for some this can turn into a chronic or recurrent problem. For these patients, treatment is aimed at nonoperative modalities.

Bed rest is to be avoided, multiple studies show that staying active results in improvement of both chronic and acute low back pain [5–7]. NSAIDS and COX-2 inhibitors have been shown to improve back pain in both the acute and chronic setting [8, 9]. NSAIDs and acetaminophen have also been found to be equivalent in managing back pain [7]. Other modalities, such as traction, physical therapy, lumbar supports, and behavioral therapy, have not been shown to be more effective than placebo for back pain. For this reason, it is recommended that during episodes of back pain without radiculopathic symptoms, the masters athlete remains active and uses NSAIDs or acetaminophen as needed. With rare exception, the masters athlete should not be held out of sport as a result of back pain.

Spinal Stenosis

Spinal stenosis is a disease process in which neurologic structures have limited space, either as a result of degenerative changes, congenital anomalies, or traumatic events. For the purposes of the masters athlete, degenerative changes are the major causes of spinal stenosis. Both bony anatomy and soft tissues contribute to these phenomena. Facet osteophytes, uncinate spurs, and spondylolisthesis can create canal stenosis in patients. Herniation of discs, synovial facet cysts, and anomalies of the ligamentum flavum are soft tissue causes of canal stenosis. It is important for the physician to understand that while each of these causes is separate, they often can occur together further exacerbating symptoms. While back and buttock pain may be the presenting symptom, the most common indication for intervention and treatment is neurogenic claudication. Neurogenic claudication is defined by fatigue in the muscles as a result of compression of neural elements.

Many patients with spinal stenosis are asymptomatic. In a symptomatic patient with spinal stenosis, the cardinal finding is improvement of neurogenic claudication with flexion of the spine.

In deciding on treatment for spinal stenosis, the SPORT trial has shown that patients with neurologic symptoms did better at 4-year follow-up with surgical decompression with and without fusion as compared to patients undergoing nonoperative modalities [10]. Patients without neurologic symptoms therefore are poor surgical candidates, and nonoperative modalities should be employed. In looking at return to play, there is considerable debate as to when patients should return to sport and even whether they should. In patients requiring lumbar fusion, it is generally thought that patients in a sport requiring hyperextension or high compressive loads should be counseled that it is not generally recommended to go back to the sport; however patients engaging in sports that do not need the ability to hyperextend or high compressive loads may generally return to sport as tolerated, but however must be counseled that they may not be able to perform at the same level as their pre-injury state.

Intervertebral Disc Disease

Intervertebral discs in the spine are responsible for spinal motion and stability in the spine. Discs are composed of two layers—the annulus fibrosis and the nucleus pulposus. The annulus fibrosus is the outer structure that surrounds the nucleus pulposus. The annulus fibrosus is composed primarily of type 1 collagen as opposed to the type 2 collagen in the nucleus pulposus. Both portions of the disc are composed of water and proteoglycans. The annulus fibrosus provides tensile strength, while the nucleus pulposus provides compressibility to the disc. Herniations occur acutely when the annulus fibrosus fails allowing the nucleus pulposus to herniate. With age this can occur with lower forces applied to the disc. This is a result of decrease in water content and conversion to fibrocartilage associate with disc aging. As discs age, there is a decrease in nutritional content, viable cells, and proteoglycans [11]. There is also an increase in lactate, degradative enzyme activity, keratin sulfate to chondroitin sulfate ratio, and density of fibroblast like cells in the annulus fibrosus [11]. These changes make the disc less amenable to tolerating stress. In the aging athlete, this can present with discogenic pain and radiculopathy.

Weiler et al. performed a histologic analysis showing that the amount of degeneration in the spine is affected by the region of the spine. This was done in patients with genetic predisposition to disc degeneration. The finding was that the lumbar intervertebral discs in a patient had more degenerative changes than the cervicothoracic region [12]. The conclusion to be drawn from this is that lumbar disc herniations should be more common in patients as opposed to cervicothoracic herniations. Incidence of cervical disc herniation in symptomatic and asymptomatic patients 60 years of age and older is 86% in men and 89% in women [13]. In the lumbar spine, it is generally agreed that there is a higher incidence of disc herniation in the geriatric population related to higher compressive load on the lumbar spine. Disc herniations tend to occur in high-mobility areas specifically in the cervical spine at C5-6 and C6-7 and the lumbar spine at L4-5 and L5-S1. Depending on the pattern of herniation, the symptoms may vary between discogenic back pain in central lesions to radiculopathic symptoms in paracentral, far lateral, and large central lesions.

Cervical Disc Herniations

Cervical disc herniations (CDH) can be treated with both surgical and nonsurgical means. Generally, radiculopathy is the presenting symptom and typically has a favorable course. Counseling patients about the natural history is an important step in managing expectations for patients. Lees et al. showed that the natural history of CDH is relatively benign. In this case series of patients, 45% had only one episode of radiculopathy, 30% had recurrent mild symptoms, and only 25% of these patients had continued or worsening symptoms. It is important to note that none of these patients progressed to myelopathy [14].

Nonoperative modalities such as soft collar use and traction do not have any evidence-based support for efficacy and thus cannot be recommended by the authors [15, 16]. There is data suggesting that a short course of oral corticosteroids can improve patient function and pain [17]. Epidural steroid injections have also been shown to give patients pain relief when compared to local injections [18]. As a result, corticosteroids are routinely used in initial management of cervical radiculopathy. Interestingly, physical therapy is often prescribed for initial treatment in patients with CDH. This is in spite of sparse data showing any change in symptoms when compared to the natural history. When nonoperative modalities fail, surgical options can be explored. Treatment options include anterior cervical discectomy and fusion (ACDF), cervical disc arthroplasty (CDA), and posterior foraminotomy.

ACDF is considered the treatment of choice, in which all disc material is removed and the vertebrae are fused together. This method allows the surgeon to decompress the nerves but also correct any kyphosis in the cervical region. Often, structural allograft or a cage can be used in the intervertebral disc space to both aid in fusion and correct deformity with both having equivalent outcomes [19]. There is controversy as to whether an anterior plate is needed when treating single-level disease. However multiple studies show improved outcomes when an anterior plate is used in these scenarios [20, 21].If plates are not used, there is a risk of pseudoarthrosis, increased kyphosis, and even catastrophic graft migration.

The anterior approach to the cervical spine can put the recurrent laryngeal nerve at risk. In patients that have had prior radiation, surgery, or infection, this can greatly increase the risk. Some studies show this risk to be as high as 25%. The injury can range from local ischemia and neuropraxia to transection and in most cases without transection resolves in 3 months. With this in mind, it is important to recognize that the surgeon can use a posterior approach to potentially avoid these complications [22, 23].

Posterior cervical laminoforaminotomy is an accepted technique to decompress the cervical spine in patients with cervical radiculopathy. By utilizing this technique, the nerve root is directly decompressed. This technique has the added benefit that fusion is not always indicated as the facet is often not violated. In the aging patient, bony obstruction of the foramina may necessitate violation of the facet which would force the surgeon to fuse that level. Outcomes for this procedure are the same for ACDF. In a study of 33 patients undergoing either ACDF or posterior laminoforaminotomy, patients had 95 and 75% satisfaction, respectively, at 4.2 years follow-up [24]. The major complaint after this approach is neck pain which is typically related to muscle dissection. Data suggests that both ACDF and posterior laminoforaminotomy are acceptable treatments for cervical disc herniation.

CDA is a relatively new method of surgical treatment for cervical disc herniation. This method allows the patient to maintain their motion as opposed to a fusion. Studies show that outcomes of CDA are equivalent to ACDF [25]. There is some thought that this method of treatment may also limit adjacent segment disease in patients; however this has not been borne out in the literature [20]. A major limitation in determining the efficacy of this new modality is that many studies have significant industry support. At this time the authors cannot recommend for or against this treatment modality.

Return to play after surgical intervention depends on the extent and type of surgery. In posterior laminoforaminotomy, it is generally agreed that patients can return to play after recovery from surgery. If two or more levels are decompressed posteriorly, then return to play is not advisable. ACDF patients with one level fusion can safely return to sport. Two level fusions depend on the patient's goals and the sport played. In contact sports, it is typically thought to be a relative contraindication. In three or more level fusion, return to sport is contraindicated as the range of motion is greatly reduced. When counseling patients about return to play, it is important to manage expectations. Hsu et al. showed that players in the NFL that had CDH, regardless of operative versus nonoperative intervention, were able to return to sport at the same level pre-injury. However, athletes that underwent operative intervention had a higher rate of return to sport. In the masters athlete, it must be stressed that they may not have the same performance after this injury and that they should keep this in mind when deciding about returning to play.

Lumbar Disc Herniations

Lumbar disc herniation can present with a variety of symptoms, from discogenic back pain to radiculopathy and even cauda equina syndrome. The natural history of these herniations is typically favorable. Patients treated with a corset and bed rest have 80% recovery at 6 weeks, 90% recovery at 12 weeks, and 93% recovery at 24 weeks [26]. Furthermore the study by Hakelius did not show a difference in recovery with surgery when looking at patients with stable motor deficits. Typically patients will have symptoms but often they resolve even without treatment. If treatment is necessary, there are a variety of nonoperative modalities at the physicians' disposal.

Indications for nonoperative therapy are the absence of progressive neurologic deficit and the absence of cauda equine syndrome. Patients that do well with nonoperative management clinically have the absence of leg pain with spinal extension, absence of stenosis on imaging, and resolution of deficits within 12 weeks [27]. Patients that are physically fit and educated generally do well with nonoperative treatment [27]. Workers compensation and psychologic maladies are associated with poor outcomes with nonoperative treatment [27]. Treatment modalities include medication, epidural steroid injections, and physical therapy.

Physical therapy is a commonly used modality for treating LDH. However, there are no studies that show that it significantly affects the natural history of LDH. While it does have a role in axial back pain, it is unclear if it is any better than having patients continue activities of daily living [28].

Medical management of lumbar disc herniation includes nonsteroidal anti-inflammatory drugs (NSAIDs), corticosteroids, and antiepileptics. The data on NSAIDs shows that there is no benefit for radiculopathic pain [29]. Corticosteroids are commonly given to patients with radiculopathy; however studies show that they are not more effective than a placebo pill in treating lumbosacral radiculopathy [30]. Lastly, antiepileptics such as gabapentin are commonly used to treat pain. There is no study showing that this is effective for patients; however lamotrigine has been showing to improve radiculopathic symptoms [31].

Epidural steroid injections (ESI) have long been used for treatment of lumbar radiculopathy. Historically, it has been shown that ESI is beneficial to pain control and function in the short term in the treatment of acute radiculopathy [29]. There are multiple techniques for ESI, but the two most common approaches are inter-laminar and transforaminal. Interlaminar injections deliver steroid to the anterior epidural space. The downside is that this may not necessarily change the outcomes for patients likely related to the amount of dispersion with this technique. In fact, studies show that this technique offers on average 3 weeks of improved neurologic symptoms but does not offer sustained benefit in patient outcomes including avoidance of surgical intervention [32]. Transforaminal injections puts steroid directly around the affected nerve. Studies show that the transforaminal injection is better at reducing pain score and preventing the need for surgery in patients with LDH [33]. Epidural steroid injections are a viable option for controlling patient's symptoms; however the data available suggests it does not significantly affect the natural history.

When conservative therapy fails, surgical decompression becomes a viable option. In patients with progressive neurologic symptoms or cauda equina syndrome, it is agreed that surgical management is more reliable for resolving symptoms. However, patients with stable neurologic symptoms studies show no benefit to surgical management as opposed to conservative management [34]. There are three main methods of decompression—the traditional laminotomy-discectomy, endoscopic discectomy, and microdiscectomy. No study shows that any of these are superior to the others.

Interestingly, data shows that the size of the disc does not predict failure of nonsurgical treatment. In fact, studies show larger discs are more likely to spontaneously resolve [35]. In a similar vein, there is some question as to how much disc should be removed. Studies show that there is no benefit to removing more disc and that in fact it may contribute to back pain in patients over time [36]. With regard to outcomes, patients with psychosocial issues and worse self-described health status as measured by the SF-36 have worse outcomes with surgery [37]. It is imperative that expectations after surgery are thoroughly discussed before proceeding with surgery.

When considering surgery, it is important to review the natural history of LDH with patients and try conservative therapy before proceeding to surgery. The only indication to proceed with surgery in LDH with stable neurologic symptoms is intractable radicular pain. Adherence to this tenet and patient counseling can lead to better outcomes for patients. Return to play is acceptable in LDH treated both conservatively and surgically. Hsu et al. have shown that the rate of return to play with LDH is the same across both nonoperative and operative groups, with age being shown to be a negative predictor for the number of games played [38]. In counseling the masters athlete, it is thus important to make sure to temper expectations with regard to returning to play at the same level, while they may be able to return to play, they may not be able to participate in their sport at the same level.

References

1. Leboeuf-Yde C, Lauritsen JM. The prevalence of low back pain in the literature. A structured review of 26 Nordic studies from 1954 to 1993. Spine. 1995;20:2112–8.
2. WHO. The burden of musculoskeletal conditions at the start of the new millennium. In: World Health Organization technical report series. 2003.
3. Heneweer H, Staes F, Aufdemkampe G, et al. Physical activity and low back pain: a systematic review of recent literature. Eur Spine J. 2011;20:826–45.
4. Heneweer H, Vanhees L, Picavet HS. Physical activity and low back pain: a U-shaped relation? Pain. 2009;143:21–5.
5. Malmivaara A, Häkkinen U, Aro T, Heinrichs M-L, Koskenniemi L, Kuosma E, Lappi S, Paloheimo R, Servo C, Vaaranen V, Hernberg S. The treatment of acute low back pain—bed rest, exercises, or ordinary activity. N Engl J Med. 1995;332(6):351–5.
6. Rozenberg S, Delval C, Rezvani Y. Bed rest or normal activity for patients with acute low back pain: a randomized controlled trial. Spine. 2002;27:1487–93.
7. Wiesel SW, Cuckler JM, Deluca F, Jones F, Zeide MS, Rothman RH. Acute low back pain: an objective analysis of conservative therapy. Spine. 1980;5:324–30.
8. Berry H, Bloom B, Hamilton EBD, Swinson DR. Naproxen sodium, diflunisal, and placebo in the treatment of chronic back pain. Ann Rheum Dis. 1982;41:129–32.
9. Babej-Dolle R, Freytag S, Eckmeyer J, Zerle G, Schinzel S, Schmeider G, Stankov G. Parenteral dipyrone versus diclofenac and placebo in patients with acute lumbago or sciatic pain: randomized observer-blind multicenter study. Int J Clin Pharmacol Ther. 1994;32:204–9.
10. Weinstein JN, Tosteson TD, Lurie JD, Tosteson A, Blood E, Herkowitz H, Cammisa F, Albert T, Boden SD, Hilibrand A, Goldberg H, Berven S, An H. Surgical versus non-operative treatment for lumbar spinal stenosis four year results of the Spine Patient Outcomes Research Trial (SPORT). Spine. 2010;35:1329–38.
11. Boos N, Weissbach S, Rohrbach H, Weiler C, Spratt KF, Nerlich AG. Classification of age-related changes in lumbar intervertebral discs: 2002 Volvo Award in basic science. Spine. 2002;27(23):2631–44.
12. Weiler C, Schietzsch M, Kirchner T, Nerlich AG, Boos N, Wuertz K. Age-related changes in human cervical, thoracal and lumbar intervertebral disc exhibit a strong intra-individual correlation. Eur Spine J. 2012;21(Suppl 6):S810–8.
13. Matsumoto M, Fujimura Y, Suzuki N, et al. MRI of cervical intervertebral discs in asymptomatic subjects. J Bone Joint Surg Br. 1998;80(1):19–24.
14. Lees F, Turner JW. Natural history and prognosis of cervical spondylosis. Br Med J. 1963;2:1607–10.
15. Naylor JR, Mulley GP. Surgical collars: a survey of their prescription and use. Br J Rheumatol. 1991;30:282–4.
16. Swezey RL, Swezey AM, Warner K. Efficacy of home cervical traction therapy. Am J Phys Med Rehabil. 1999;78:30–2.
17. Ghasemi M, Masaeli A, Rezvani M, Shaygannejad V, Golabchi K, Norouzi R. Oral prednisolone in the treatment of cervical radiculopathy: a randomized placebo controlled trial. J Res Med Sci. 2013;18(Suppl 1):S43–6.
18. Stav A, Ovadia L, Sternberg A, et al. Cervical epidural steroid injection for cervicobrachialgia. Acta Anaesthesiol Scand. 1993;37:562–6.

19. Barlocher CB, Barth A, Krauss JK, Binggeli R, Seiler RW. Comparative evaluation of microd-iscectomy only, autograft fusion, polymethylmethacrylate interposition, and threaded titanium cage fusion for treatment of single-level cervical disc disease: a prospective randomized study in 125 patients. Neurosurg Focus. 2002;12(1):E4.
20. Jawahar A, Cavanaugh DA, Kerr EJ 3rd, Birdsong EM, Nunley PD. Total disc arthroplasty does not affect the incidence of adjacent segment degeneration in cervical spine: results of 93 patients in three prospective randomized clinical trials. Spine J. 2010;10(12):1043–8.
21. Song KJ, Choi BW, Kim GH, Song JH. Usefulness of polyetheretherketone (PEEK) cage with plate augmentation for anterior arthrodesis in traumatic cervical spine injury. Spine J. 2010;10(1):50–7.
22. Watters WC 3rd, Levinthal R. Anterior cervical discectomy with and without fusion. Results, complications, and long-term follow-up. Spine (Phila Pa 1976). 1994;19(20):2343–7.
23. Bohlman HH, Emery SE, Goodfellow DB, Jones PK. Robinson anterior cervical discectomy and arthrodesis for cervical radiculopathy. Long-term follow-up of one hundred and twenty-two patients. J Bone Joint Surg Am. 1993;75(9):1298–307.
24. Herkowitz HN, Kurz LT, Overholt DP. Surgical management of cervical soft disc herniation. A comparison between the anterior and posterior approach. Spine (Phila Pa 1976). 1990;15(10):1026–30.
25. Coric D, Nunley PD, Guyer RD, et al. Prospective, randomized, multicenter study of cervical arthroplasty: 269 patients from the KineflexIC artificial disc investigational device exemption study with a minimum 2-year follow-up. J Neurosurg Spine. 2011;15(4):348–58.
26. Hakelius A. Prognosis in sciatica. A clinical follow-up of surgical and non-surgical treatment. Acta Orthop Scand Suppl. 1970;129:1–76.
27. Githens PB, O'Conner T, Weil U, Calogero JA, Holford TR, White AA 3rd, Walter SD, Ostfeld AM, Southwick WO. Acute prolapsed lumbar intervertebral disc. An epidemiologic study with special reference to driving automobiles and cigarette smoking. Spine. 1984;9:608–13.
28. Hofstee DJ, Gijtenbeek JM, Hoogland PH, van Houwelingen HC, Kloet A, Lotters F, Tans JT. Westeinde sciatica trial: randomized controlled study of bed rest and physiotherapy for acute sciatica. J Neurosurg. 2002;96(1 Suppl):45–9.
29. Vroomen PC, de Krom MC, Slofstra PD, Knottnerus JA. Conservative treatment of sciatica: a systematic review. J Spinal Disord. 2000;13:463–9.
30. Beresford HR. Dexamethasone is not superior to placebo for treating lumbosacral radicular pain. Neurology. 1986;36:1593–4.
31. Damunni G, Hoffer E, Baum Y, Krivoy N. Lamotrigine for intractable sciatica: correlation between dose, plasma concentration and analgesia. Eur J Pain. 2003;7:485–91.
32. Arden NK, Price C, Reading I, Stubbing J, Hazelgrove J, Dunne C, Michel M, Rogers P, Cooper C, WEST Study Group. A multicentre randomized controlled trial of epidural cortico-steroid injections for sciatica: the WEST study. Rheumatology (Oxford). 2005;44:1399–406.
33. Schaufele M, Hatch L. Interlaminar versus transforaminal epidural injections in the treatment of symptomatic lumbar intervertebral disc herniations. Arch Phys Med Rehabil. 2002;83:1661.
34. Dubourg G, Rozenberg S, Fautrel B, Valls-Bellec I, Bissery A, Lang T, Faillot T, Duplan B, Briancon D, Levy-Weil F, Morlock G, Crouzet J, Gatfosse M, Bonnet C, Houvenagel E, Hary S, Brocq O, Poiraudeau S, Beaudreuil J, de Sauverzac C, Durieux S, Levade MH, Esposito P, Maitrot D, Goupille P, Valat JP, Bourgeois P. A pilot study on the recovery from paresis after lumbar disc herniation. Spine. 2002;27:1426–31.
35. Bush K, Cowan N, Katz DE, Gishen P. The natural history of sciatica associated with disc pathology. A prospective study with clinical and independent radiologic follow-up. Spine. 1992;17:1205–12.
36. Balderston RA, Gilyard GG, Jones AA, Wiesel SW, Spengler DM, Bigos SJ, Rothman RH. The treatment of lumbar disc herniation: simple fragment excision versus disc space curettage. J Spinal Disord. 1991;4:22–5.

37. Slover J, Abdu WA, Hanscom B, Lurie J, Weinstein JN. Can condition-specific health surveys be specific to spine disease? An analysis of the effect of comorbidities on baseline condition-specific and general health survey scores. Spine. 2006;31:125–71.
38. Hsu WK, Mccarthy KJ, Savage JW, et al. The Professional Athlete Spine Initiative: outcomes after lumbar disc herniation in 342 elite professional athletes. Spine J. 2011;11(3):180–6.

Part III
Thriving as a Masters Athlete

Chapter 14
Return to Sport Following Total Joint Arthroplasty

Michael J. O'Malley and Brian A. Klatt

Introduction

Total hip and knee arthroplasties are two of the most successful procedures. Both have been found to be cost-effective and beneficial to a patient's quality of life [1–4]. Historically, joint arthroplasty was reserved for those above the age of 65 who were debilitated from the pain of end-stage osteoarthritis. However, as the success of the operation has become widely known, patients are often inquiring about joint replacement earlier to help maintain and/or restore activity including athletic participation. The young active patient with end-stage osteoarthritis is in a therapeutic dilemma. The mechanism of failure for the majority of lower extremity joint replacements at long-term follow-up is aseptic loosening [5]. There is obvious concern that joint arthroplasty in young patients would therefore succumb to wear earlier due to increased use, potentially condemning the patient to numerous revisions and potentially catastrophic failure in their lifetime [6–10]. Despite such concern, arthroplasty is used to treat end-stage osteoarthritis in younger patients that seek to restore function and even return to athletic activity [11, 12]. Fortunately, the concern for increased wear and early failure has not been fully realized, and survival rates as high as 94% can be found at nearly 20 years in young active patients [12]. In this chapter we will explore the literature and current recommendations concerning hip and knee arthroplasties in patients that wish to remain physically active in sports.

M. J. O'Malley, MD · B. A. Klatt, MD (✉)
Department of Orthopaedic Surgery, University of Pittsburgh Medical Center (UPMC), Pittsburgh, PA, USA
e-mail: omalleymj3@upmc.edu; klattba@upmc.edu

© Springer International Publishing AG, part of Springer Nature 2018   167
V. J. Wright, K. K. Middleton (eds.), *Masterful Care of the Aging Athlete*,
https://doi.org/10.1007/978-3-319-16223-2_14

Total Hip Arthroplasty

Implant Design and Outcomes

Sir John Charnley invented the modern total hip arthroplasty (THA) in the early 1960s. Today more than one million hip replacements are performed each year worldwide, with a projected increase to 3.5 million by 2030 [13]. Hip arthroplasty, an incredibly successful operation, has even been named the "operation of the century" in a review article published by Lancet [14].

Sir John Charnley's low friction-arthroplasty consisted of a monoblock polished stainless steel stem and a polyethylene liner, both of which were secured to the bone by polymethyl methacrylate bone cement [15]. Charnley's results were revolutionary with early results demonstrating >90% survival at 10 years and 78% at 35 years [16, 17]. There were concerns in the United States that fixation of the prosthesis with bone cement was less favorable in younger patients, and this leads to a surge in the development of cementless implants [18–22]. Over the years the development of cementless implants has dominated the US market especially in younger, more active patients. The proposed benefits of cementless implants include the capacity for bone remodeling in response to stress while preserving attachment in the bone [19, 23].

In the 1990s a phenomenon of profound osteolysis and aseptic loosening from a macrophage-mediated inflammatory response to microscopic wear particles generated from the metal on polyethylene articulation was realized [24, 25]. The lysis caused severe bone loss and failure of components especially in young active patients. This resulted in a surge of interest in alternative bearing surfaces such at ceramics and metal on metal (MOM) as well as alternative forms of replacement such as hip resurfacing. Unfortunately each of these bearing and implant options had other problems, and their utilization has dramatically decreased [26, 27].

It was determined that the cause of early polyethylene wear was related to oxidation of the polyethylene during the sterilization process [24, 28]. Irradiation of polyethylene during sterilization results in cleavage of the polyethylene chain leading to the production of free radicals. In the presence of oxygen, these free radicals become oxidized, leading to decreased fatigue strength and increased brittleness of the polyethylene resulting in poor wear characteristics. Interestingly, it was found that if polyethylene was irradiated in an inert atmosphere, the free radical chains could bond to other free radicals on adjacent chains resulting in cross-linking between polyethylene chains. This technique has been shown to greatly increase wear resistance [29].

The most recent literature shows negligible polyethylene wear at 10 years [30, 31]. A multicenter study published in 2012 sought to compare the wear rate of a new electron beam irradiated highly cross-linked polyethylene (HXLPE) to historic controls at 7- and 10-year follow-up. The authors included 768 THA patients and found significantly lower wear rates in the HXLPE patients compared to historic controls at 7 and 10 years. There was no evidence of osteolysis or cases of revision for aseptic loosening in the HXLPE group [32]. Improved biomaterials, methods of component fixation, and increased longevity of the prosthesis have led to a more confident expansion of arthroplasty indications to the younger and more active patient.

Indications

Prior to the development of the total hip replacement, treatments for end-stage osteoarthritis were Girdlestone hip resection or an arthrodesis. At its conception, the THA was considered a salvage procedure until it could be proven effective. Historically, total hip arthroplasty was reserved for those over the age of 65 and in whom the pain of osteoarthritis was debilitating. The objective of the procedure was principally pain relief. The anticipated demands on implants were very low with most patients expecting the ability to comfortably perform activities of daily living. Today, the main indication for THA remains pain and dysfunction related to end-stage hip arthrosis that is refractory to nonoperative measures. However, as described above, with the advent of improved implants, bearing surfaces, and surgical technique, surgeons are becoming more confident and willing to implant hip replacements in younger patients with higher expectations of functional return.

Return to Athletic Activity

To the authors' knowledge, there are no prospective randomized studies evaluating the safety and ability to return to sport following total hip arthroplasty. When discussing return to activity or return to sports with postoperative hip patients, there are several questions that need to be answered. *What percentages of patients are able to return to athletic activity following total hip arthroplasty? Are there predictors that determine which patients are more likely to return to sport? Which sports are people able to return to, and do they change their activity postoperatively? When can patients return to athletic activity? What are the surgeons' recommendations regarding return to sport?*

Several recent studies have tried to determine the percentage of patients that are able to return to athletic activity following hip replacement and which factors are predictive of return [33–37]. There is significant variability in the study designs, patient populations included, and outcome measures. The range of patients that return to athletic activity postoperatively as documented in the literature is 61–100%. Several studies show an increase in percentage of patients participating in athletic activity following hip replacement, while others show a decrease [33, 34, 36, 37]. A longitudinal multicenter study published by Hoch et al. showed an increase in the number of active patients postoperatively (52% from 36%) and remained active for at least 1 h a week at 5 years following THA [34]. Additionally Chatterji et al. retrospectively reviewed the activity of 216 patients (235 hips) that underwent THA [33]. They found that participation in sport increased from 188 to

196 patients. Subjectively, patients reported that surgery had a beneficial effect on their athletic performance; however, the number of sporting activities decreased from an average of 1.9 per patient to 1.7 (10%). Specific activities that showed increased participation were walking and water aerobics. In contrast, golf, tennis, and jogging had a significant decrease in number of participants. Tennis and jogging lost nearly all participation, 13 out of 14 and 6 out of 7 patients, respectively [33]. Other studies have similarly shown a decrease in high-impact activities following hip arthroplasty [34, 37].

Williams et al. published a study using a validated activity questionnaire (UCLA activity score) to evaluate the intensity of activity that patients participate in following arthroplasty [36]. They retrospectively reviewed 735 patients who underwent a variety of primary and revision arthroplasties of the hip and knee and investigated their postoperative activity profile as well as explored predictors of participation in sports. The UCLA activity score ranges from 1 to 10, where 1 signifies inactive and dependent on others and 10 is participation in high-impact sports such as jogging and tennis. A score of 7 and above is defined as returning to intense activity. In this study, all patients had a significant increase in UCLA score from pre- to postop. Preoperatively 91 patients (12.3%) had a score of 7 or more, which increased to 274 patients (37.2%) postoperatively (16.6% vs. 43.3% specific to THA). Preop UCLA activity score, younger patients, male sex, and body mass index independently predicted a UCLA score of 7 or more postoperatively [36]. Other studies have similarly shown that younger age and male gender are predictive of postoperative participation in athletic activity [34, 37].

There are several reasons why patients may not return to athletic activity postoperatively. Foremost, there is significant variability in surgeon recommendations regarding permitted activities postoperatively. Many surgeons are reluctant to release patients to unrestricted high-intensity activity [37, 38]. Additionally, patients may have self-imposed precautions based on their own concerns. The two most common self-reported reasons for inability to return to sport following hip replacement were precaution (53%) and pain elsewhere in the body (26%) [34].

Though many surgeons recommend against high-impact activities following hip replacement, the question remains as to the capability of patients to return such sports. Furthermore, are those patients able to return to a high level of competitive play? Mont et al. sought to investigate by sending a questionnaire to United States Tennis Association members to identify patients who had undergone hip replacement. Fifty men and eight women responded (75 hips). The average age of the respondent was 70 years old (average age at surgery, 62). The authors reported that 100% of patients were satisfied with the result and were able to obtain a level of play that was at or near their presymptomatic level. Three patients required revision (4%), which was not significantly different from the general population. However, because of the selection bias present in this study, the authors caution that no conclusion should be drawn concerning revision rates after high-impact activities such as tennis [39].

There is biomechanical literature describing hip forces during walking, running, and alpine and cross-country skiing in native hips [40]. Using an accelerometer the authors were able to determine peak hip joint contact forces during each activity.

Walking resulted in peak joint contact forces at 2.5 times body weight (BW), while running was 5.2 BW. During alpine skiing the joint forces varied based on skiing conditions. They ranged from 4.1 during long turns on flat slopes to 7.8 BW on short radius turns on steep slopes. Cross-country skiing was around 4 BW, between walking and running (van Der). To the authors' knowledge, there are no mechanical studies evaluating the effects of these activities on a hip prosthesis.

However, Gschwend et al. from Sweden conducted a retrospective cohort study of 2 groups of 50 THA patients in which one is active in skiing (Group A) and the other not (Group B) and followed them for 5–10 years [41]. The authors found that at 5 years there were no signs of loosening in the skiing group, whereas five patients in the inactive group had radiographic evidence of loosening ($p < 0.05$). At 10 years, however, there were two cases of loosening in Group A and none in Group B. Additionally there was a higher wear rated noted in the skiing group 2.1 mm vs. 1.5 mm ($p < 0.05$) though the amount of osteolysis was not different between groups. The functional scores were higher in Group A at 10-year follow-up ($p < 0.001$). Though this data suggests skiing may increase the rate of wear as compared to inactive controls, it should be noted that the patients in Group A were not specifically active in only skiing, and many were active year round. The authors of this study do not restrict the experienced skier from the psychological and cardiovascular benefits obtained by skiing but do admit that more negative long-term effects may be seen due to increased wear.

Another popular sport is golf. Mallon and Callaghan evaluated 115 amateur golfers at an average of 6 years following hip replacement [35]. The authors reported that all patients who played golf preoperatively returned to playing golf postoperatively. Eighty-seven percent of the golfers reported no hip pain while playing golf postoperatively. The average handicap increased by 1.1 strokes, and the average drive length increased by 3.3 yards. Other studies have shown patients are able to return to judo, gymnastics, and soccer [6, 34, 42].

Hip Resurfacing vs. THA

Early in the 2000s, there was a surge of interest in hip resurfacing (HR) around the world. In the United Kingdom, resurfacing accounted for 46% of all hip replacements done in patients younger than 55 [26]. The purported advantages over THA include increased survival, less invasive, easier to revise, and superior functional outcome. These claims have not been fully supported in the literature, and in fact several populations of patients have been found to do worse. These include women, small femoral heads, developmental dysplasia of the hip, older patients, and certain implant designs [26]. Additionally the complications of metal-on-metal articulations have also been seen in hip resurfacing [26, 43, 44]. Despite this there remains interest from both patients and surgeons in hip resurfacing.

Banerjee et al. sought to evaluate the level of sports activity following hip resurfacing [6]. Preoperatively, 98% of patients participated in sporting activities, and of those, 98% returned to sport postoperatively. As noted following THA, there was a significant decrease in the number of sporting activities participated (3.6–3.2). There was also a shift toward lower-intensity sport disciplines like cycling, walking, and weight training, whereas high-impact sports such as tennis, jogging, soccer, squash, and volleyball had a significant decrease in participation. Overall patients exhibited an increase in physical activity post-operatively based on the Grimby scale. Williams et al. did not find a difference between THA and HR in regard to return to high-level activity postoperatively [36].

Authors' Recommendations

This is a topic that is very difficult to design and perform a high-quality prospective, randomized controlled trial to determine the ability of patients to return to sport as well as short- and long-term effects on survival of the prosthesis. As described above there are several shortcomings in the literature available for review. The studies are mostly retrospective and cross-sectional, involving questionnaires that are often not validated. Few studies presented in this chapter use follow-up radiographs to look for wear or osteolysis related to increased activity. The patient populations included in the studies are also inconsistent, and the authors do not consistently define the level of activity present preoperatively or the intensity postoperatively. There is significant age variation between studies, with most studies containing patients >65 years old making an extrapolation to a young, active patient problematic. Due to such variation and lack of high-quality studies to guide surgeon recommendations, we must rely on expert opinion.

In 2007 Klein et al. published consensus guidelines on return to athletic activity after total hip arthroplasty based on a survey of the Hip Society (HS) and American Association of Hip and Knee Surgeons (AAHKS) [45]. The survey listed 37 sports activities for which the surgeons were asked to classify their recommendation for a standard (metal-on-polyethylene) THA into one of four categories: allow, allow with experience, not allowed, or undecided. The response rate was 93% for the Hip Society and 72% for AAHKS. The list of activities and recommendations are found in Table 14.1. The activity recommendations varied between the two societies with regard to stair climber, doubles tennis, weight machines, and rowing. These activities were allowed with experience by the Hip Society but were allowed regardless by the members of AAHKS. Snowboarding was not allowed by the HS and undecided by the AAHKS members. The 17 activities that were given an allow recommendation received an average of 84% of votes (range 60–99%). Racquetball/squash, baseball/softball, and snowboarding were the activities with the most votes for not allow (60, 57, and 55%, respectively).

In our practice the indications for total hip arthroplasty remain pain and dysfunction related to end-stage hip arthrosis that is refractory to nonoperative management including activity modification and nonsteroidal anti-inflammatory medications. The standard bearing surface used for all patients is ceramic-on-highly cross-linked

Table 14.1 Consensus guidelines for return to activities by the members of HS and AAHKS

Allow	Allow with experience	Not allowed	Undecided
Golf	Downhill skiing	Racquetball/squash	Martial arts
Swimming	Cross-country skiing	Jogging	Singles tennis
Doubles tennis	Weight lifting	Contact sports (football, basketball, soccer)	
Stair climber	Ice skating/ rollerblading	High-impact aerobics	
Walking	Pilates	Baseball/softball	
Speed walking		Snowboarding	
Hiking			
Stationary skiing			
Bowling			
Treadmill			
Road cycling			
Stationary bicycling			
Elliptical			
Low-impact aerobics			
Rowing			
Dancing (ballroom, jazz, square)			
Weight machines			

Reproduced with permission from Kline et al. Return to Athletic Activity after Total Hip Arthroplasty, The Journal of Arthroplasty 22(2) 2007

polyethylene. In our practice, the general consensus for duration before return to athletic activity was 3–6 months. Most surgeons in our practice recommend against repetitive high-impact activities such as basketball and jogging. All surgeons allow tennis, downhill skiing, cycling, and golf. The case of metal-on-metal bearings deserves a special note. We would allow high-impact activities in a patient with a well-functioning metal on metal joint, but this bearing is no longer implanted at our institution. The risks of catastrophic failure outweigh the benefits of using these joints in our practice.

Total Knee Arthroplasty

Indications

The primary indications for total knee arthroplasty have historically been pain, deformity, loss of motion, and functional impairment that is recalcitrant to nonoperative measures. Though these indications remain unchanged today, patients' expectations have evolved, from pure pain relief to functional improvement, which often includes the ability to return to sport [46]. Patients are presenting to the surgeon after the earliest signs of dysfunction, seeking surgery to restore their level of pre-arthritis activity.

Implant Design

The two most common knee designs are posterior cruciate retaining and posterior cruciate substituting/sacrificing. In meta-analysis, no difference has been found in survival at long-term follow-up between designs [47, 48]. It is likely that the most important aspect of the procedure is the restoration of the joint line and mechanical alignment. Increased wear has been documented when alignment has not been restored to within 3° of mechanical axis [49, 50].

Modern primary total knee arthroplasty designs come in varying degree of constraint to resist deformity. Most surgeons rely on minimal constraint within the implant and instead balance the native medial and lateral ligamentous structures about the knee to restore more normal knee kinematics. Minimal constraint decreases the forces on the implants' cement/bone interface however does allow for some movement at the tibial polyethylene insert and the femoral component interface.

The conformity between the polyethylene surface and femoral component varies from manufacturer as well as design. In general, cruciate-retaining knees have less conformity at the polyethylene surface to allow for rollback of the femoral component. Posterior stabilized and mobile-bearing prostheses have increasing levels of conformity between the polyethylene and the femoral component, respectively. Additionally the conformity and contact area of the polyethylene to the femoral component are different at varying degrees of knee flexion with less conformity and contact area as flexion increases. This is different from a hip replacement, which is a ball-and-socket joint, and essentially a constant level of congruency and contact area between bearing surfaces within physiologic range of motion.

Knee Biomechanics

Biomechanical studies have evaluated the forces on the native knee during different athletic activities. Walking on level ground can produce forces three to four times that of body weight (BW), whereas walking downhill can be as high as 8 BW. Cycling has demonstrated compressive loads of 1.2 BW [51]. Using this information the authors conducted a study estimating the peak loads and contact area on total knee implants during these activities.

Kuster et al. placed three different knee designs (flat, curved, and mobile-bearing tibial inlays) in a material testing system [52]. Using Fuji pressure-sensitive film to measure the load and contact between the femoral component and polyethylene during the simulated activities (cycling, power walking, downhill walking, and jogging), the authors found that downhill walking and jogging resulted in the largest contact area with peak loads above the yield point of the polyethylene. Furthermore, the peak loads occurred between 40 and 60° of knee flexion, where conformity is decreased, potentially increasing the chance of damage to the polyethylene. Power walking and cycling had the two smallest contact areas with forces that were measured above the yield point. The authors concluded that jogging and downhill hiking should be avoided post-arthroplasty while cycling and powerwalking encouraged [52, 53].

Return to Athletic Activity

There are varying rates of return to athletic activity following total knee arthroplasty documented in the literature, 64–80% [34, 36, 37, 54]. As with the literature of return to sport following hip arthroplasty, there is great variability in study design and populations included specifically in regard to age and preoperative activity level.

Bradbury et al. investigated the athletic activity of 160 patients at a mean follow-up of 5 years following total knee arthroplasty [55]. Using a mailed questionnaire, he found that 79 patients, with an average age of 67, were athletically active preoperatively. The three most common activities were golf, bowling, and tennis. Following surgery, 51 patients (65%) remained active in sports. Patients were more likely to return to low-impact activities such as bowling (92%) as compared to high-impact tennis (20%). Several other studies have shown a decrease in sports participation postoperatively [34, 37, 54]. Chatterji et al. showed that despite a decrease in number of patients that were active postoperatively and a decrease in the number of athletic activities per patient, the patients report that surgery had a beneficial effect on their sports participation (average age 70.8 at surgery) [54]. Reported reasons in the literature for why patients did not return to sport include pain in the knee, pain in other joints, medical advice, and concern for the joint [34, 37, 56]. Pain in the operative knee has been listed as the most common reason [34].

Dahm et al. published one of the largest series in the literature utilizing validated patient-reported activity levels after total knee arthroplasty at a mean 5.7 years postop [56]. One thousand two hundred and six patients responded with a 74% response rate. The average age of the patients was 67 at the time of surgery (73 at the time of survey). The authors used the UCLA activity rating survey to quantify the intensity of activities performed. The average UCLA activity rating was 7.1 (regularly participate in active events, e.g., bicycling). Men, age ≤ 70, and BMI <30 kg/m² were predictive of higher activity scores. In a similar study including a variety of hip and knee arthroplasties, Williams et al. found in addition to the ones listed above high preoperative UCLA activity rating was predictive of a score ≥ 7 postop [36].

Golf is one of the most popular athletic activities among masters athletes [57]. Many patients choose to have a knee replacement in order to continue to play. Most patients and surgeons consider it a low-impact exercise and value such benefits that allow patients to remain social, active, and outdoors. Rates of return to golf are variable in the literature [34, 37, 58, 59]. Of patients that return to play, Mallon and Callaghan stated that 16% of players report mild pain during play and 35% have a mild ache after play [59]. Active golfers saw a rise in their handicap (+4.3 strokes) and a 12-yard decrease in driving distance. Based on the current literature, golfers should be able to return to playing within 3 and 6 months with less pain than preop.

Right-handed golfers, who had a left knee replacement (target side knee), had more discomfort during play than golfers with a right knee replacement [59]. This is explained by the increased torque and rotation in the lead knee as force transfers forward during downswing and ball contact [60]. D'Lima showed that peak forces generated on the lead knee during downswing are around 4 BW, roughly the same as jogging [61]. Despite this force, most surgeons allow patients to return to golf [62].

Mont et al. analyzed the clinical and radiographic results of 31 patients (33 knees), who were identified as participating in high-impact activities on average 4 days per week [38]. The most common sports were tennis (15), jogging (9), aerobics (9), and racquetball/squash. At final follow-up the mean Knee Society score was 93 out of 100 points. Of the 33 knees, 32 were considered to have good or excellent outcome based on Knee Society score. Only one patient required revision for progressive tibial lucency.

Many of the studies presented above involve patients with an average age ≥ 65 years. The literature suggests that patients older than 60 have decreasing levels of activity; therefore it is difficult to extrapolate these results to a younger and likely more active population [56]. Conversely, the data also reveals that patients who remain active into their eighth decade can do so at a high level. In the article published by Dahm et al., 38% of patients participating in heavy manual labor or high-impact activities were greater than 70 years old [56].

To the authors' knowledge, there is a paucity of literature reporting return to athletic activity in young patients following total knee arthroplasty. Diduch et al. presented the results of 88 patients (103 knees) in patients ≤55 years old [12]. The authors found good to excellent results in all 103 knees according to the knee scores of Hospital of Special Surgery and Knee Society. Twenty-five percent of patients had a Tegner and Lysholm score of 5 indicating they were participating in high-level activities such as tennis, bicycling, skiing, or construction. The survival rate of the prosthesis was 94% at 18 years if revision of the femoral or tibial component was used as the definition of failure. It dropped to 87% if revision of the patella or polyethylene were included. These results are very encouraging for the ability to maintain a high level of activity while preserving the survival of the prosthesis.

Unicompartmental Knee Arthroplasty

Unicompartmental knee arthroplasty (UKA) involves replacing only the medial or lateral tibiofemoral compartment. The indications for UKA are more controversial than for total knee arthroplasty. Traditionally, UKA was reserved for patients older than 60, thin individuals (<180 lbs) with arthritis limited to the medial or lateral compartment of the knee and the absence of anterior knee pain [63]. Over time, proponents of UKA have refined the indications to medial or lateral disease with an intact ACL, preserved posterior bone, and fully correctable alignment, while age, weight, absence of patellofemoral disease, and anterior knee pain have been removed [64]

Survival of UKA is excellent at 10 years (98%) and has been reported as high as 91% at 20 years [65–68]. When compared to TKA, several outcome measures have been studied. Lombardi et al. found that UKA patients had better range of motion than those who had a TKA immediately postop and continued to 6 weeks [69]. UKA patients had better ROM and Knee Society scores. There was no difference in Oxford knee scores, return to work, or return to sport.

Other studies have shown better return to sport performance following UKA [58, 70]. Hopper et al. reported a 97% return to sport following UKA vs. 64% in the TKA patients ($p = 0.031$) [58]. There was a significant decrease in the number of low-impact sports performed from 1.5 preoperatively to 0.7 postoperatively, with golf and bowling losing the most participants. Additionally, return to sport was quicker in the UKA group (3.6 vs. 4.1 months).

Another partial knee arthroplasty performed is the patellofemoral arthroplasty (PFA). This is most commonly performed in women with end-stage patellofemoral disease with intact tibiofemoral compartments [71]. To the authors' knowledge, there are no studies specifically evaluating return to athletic activity or recommendations for return in the literature.

Author Recommendation

In 1999, Healy et al. published a review of athletic activity following total joint arthroplasty. The authors reported the results of a survey of the members of the Knee Society regarding their recommendations for their patients who had a knee replacement. Forty-two different activities were available to rate as allowed, allowed with experience, no opinion, or not recommended. Power analysis revealed a percentage of 73% was necessary to obtain significance. If that was not achieved, it was given the rating "no conclusion." The survey was repeated in 2005. The results of these surveys are presented in Table 14.2. High-impact exercises like volleyball, racquetball, and basketball were not recommended. As expected, low-impact exercises walking, bowling, and golf were allowed. A recommendation could not be made for downhill skiing.

Since 2005, our recommendations for activity following knee replacement have not changed much. We would prefer patients to avoid high-impact loading activities such as basketball, jogging, and volleyball. In our practice, surgeons allow patients to return to tennis and downhill skiing.

Regarding unicondylar knee replacement, we still abide by most of the original Kozin criteria when evaluating patients for a UKA. Specifically, we do not perform

Table 14.2 Results of the Knee Society survey [45]

Allowed	1999	2005	Allowed with experience	1999	2005	No consensus	1999	2005	Not recommended	1999	2005
Bowling	√	√	Canoeing	√		Square dancing	√		Baseball	√	
Stationary cycling	√	√	Road cycling	√		Fencing	√	√	Basketball	√	√
Ballroom dancing	√	√	Hiking	√		Roller skating	√	√	Football	√	√
Golf	√	√	Rowing	√	√	Downhill skiing	√		Gymnastics	√	
Horseback riding	√		Ice skating	√	√	Weight lifting	√	√	Handball	√	
Shuffleboard	√	√	Cross-country skiing	√	√	Baseball		√	Hockey	√	
Swimming	√	√	Stationary skiing	√	√	Gymnastics		√	Jogging	√	√
Normal walking	√	√	Doubles tennis	√	√	Handball		√	Rock climbing	√	
Canoeing		√	Speed walking	√		Hockey		√	Soccer	√	√
Road cycling		√	Weight machine	√		Rock climbing		√	Squash/racquetball	√	
Square dancing		√	Horseback riding		√	Squash/racquetball		√	Singles tennis	√	
Hiking		√	Downhill skiing		√	Singles tennis		√	Volleyball	√	√
Speed walking		√				Weight machine		√			

This table is constructed to accurately compare the 1999 and 2005 Knee Society surveys. The 1999 survey asked about croquet (allowed), horseshoes (allowed), shooting (allowed), and lacrosse (not recommended), which were not included in the 2005 survey. The 1999 survey asked about high-impact aerobics (not recommended) and low-impact aerobics (allowed with experience). The 2005 survey combined these activities and asked about aerobics (allowed with experience). The 2005 survey asked about yoga (allowed with experience), which was not included in the 1999 survey these procedures on overweight patients or those with severe or fixed deformity. As with a total knee replacement, the authors would recommend not returning to high-impact activities with a unicondylar knee. We do not restrict the activity of patients following UKA. For the rare patient that qualifies for a patellofemoral arthroplasty, we allow them to return to full activities without restriction.

Conclusion

Surgeons should exercise caution when performing a joint replacement with the goal to return the patient to a high level of activity. There is a generalized trend toward lower-intensity, lower-impact activity that may be patient driven, age related, or recommended by the treating surgeon. Nonetheless, it is important to council patients that they may not be able to return to a high level of activity. Furthermore, there is there is a risk for premature revision surgery due to increased wear or catastrophic failure. Some of the high-impact activities do exceed the maximum forces that the implants can withstand before failure. Prospective studies of young, active patients with long-term follow-up are necessary to accurately define the safety and capability of patients to return to high-intensity athletic activity. As implant materials, bearing surfaces, and implant fixation techniques continue to improve, we hope to use prosthetic joints that allow for high-impact activities without concern for early failure.

References

1. Laupacis A, et al. The effect of elective total hip replacement on health-related quality of life. J Bone Joint Surg Am. 1993;75(11):1619–26.
2. Chang RW, Pellisier JM, Hazen GB. A cost-effectiveness analysis of total hip arthroplasty for osteoarthritis of the hip. JAMA. 1996;275(11):858–65.
3. Jenkins PJ, et al. Predicting the cost-effectiveness of total hip and knee replacement: a health economic analysis. Bone Joint J. 2013;95-B(1):115–21.
4. Ethgen O, et al. Health-related quality of life in total hip and total knee arthroplasty. A qualitative and systematic review of the literature. J Bone Joint Surg Am. 2004;86-A(5):963–74.
5. Sadoghi P, et al. Revision surgery after total joint arthroplasty: a complication-based analysis using worldwide arthroplasty registers. J Arthroplast. 2013;28(8):1329–32.
6. Banerjee M, et al. Sports activity after total hip resurfacing. Am J Sports Med. 2010;38(6):1229–36.
7. Lavernia CJ, et al. Activity level and wear in total knee arthroplasty: a study of autopsy retrieved specimens. J Arthroplast. 2001;16(4):446–53.
8. Schmalzried TP, et al. The John Charnley Award. Wear is a function of use, not time. Clin Orthop Relat Res. 2000;381:36–46.
9. Sechriest VF 2nd, et al. Activity level in young patients with primary total hip arthroplasty: a 5-year minimum follow-up. J Arthroplast. 2007;22(1):39–47.
10. Zahiri CA, et al. Assessing activity in joint replacement patients. J Arthroplast. 1998;13(8):890–5.

11. Crowninshield RD, Rosenberg AG, Sporer SM. Changing demographics of patients with total joint replacement. Clin Orthop Relat Res. 2006;443:266–72.
12. Diduch DR, et al. Total knee replacement in young, active patients. Long-term follow-up and functional outcome. J Bone Joint Surg Am. 1997;79(4):575–82.
13. Kurtz S, et al. Projections of primary and revision hip and knee arthroplasty in the United States from 2005 to 2030. J Bone Joint Surg Am. 2007;89(4):780–5.
14. Learmonth ID, Young C, Rorabeck C. The operation of the century: total hip replacement. Lancet. 2007;370(9597):1508–19.
15. Charnley J. Total hip replacement. JAMA. 1974;230(7):1025–8.
16. Callaghan JJ, et al. Survivorship of a Charnley total hip arthroplasty. A concise follow-up, at a minimum of thirty-five years, of previous reports. J Bone Joint Surg Am. 2009;91(11):2617–21.
17. Charnley J. Total hip replacement by low-friction arthroplasty. Clin Orthop Relat Res. 1970;72:7–21.
18. Callaghan JJ, et al. Charnley total hip arthroplasty in patients less than fifty years old. A twenty to twenty-five-year follow-up note. J Bone Joint Surg Am. 1998;80(5):704–14.
19. Engh CA, Massin P. Cementless total hip arthroplasty using the anatomic medullary locking stem. Results using a survivorship analysis. Clin Orthop Relat Res. 1989;249:141–58.
20. Jones LC, Hungerford DS. Cement disease. Clin Orthop Relat Res. 1987;225:192–206.
21. Collis DK. Cemented total hip replacement in patients who are less than fifty years old. J Bone Joint Surg Am. 1984;66(3):353–9.
22. Dorr LD, Luckett M, Conaty JP. Total hip arthroplasties in patients younger than 45 years. A nine- to ten-year follow-up study. Clin Orthop Relat Res. 1990;260:215–9.
23. Engh CA, Bobyn JD. The influence of stem size and extent of porous coating on femoral bone resorption after primary cementless hip arthroplasty. Clin Orthop Relat Res. 1988;(231):7–28.
24. Norton MR, Yarlagadda R, Anderson GH. Catastrophic failure of the Elite Plus total hip replacement, with a Hylamer acetabulum and Zirconia ceramic femoral head. J Bone Joint Surg Br. 2002;84(5):631–5.
25. Stea S, et al. Behavior of Hylamer polyethylene in hip arthroplasty: comparison of two gamma sterilization techniques. Int Orthop. 2006;30(1):35–8.
26. Dunbar MJ, et al. Metal-on-metal hip surface replacement: the routine use is not justified. Bone Joint J. 2014;96-B(11 Suppl A):17–21.
27. Rajpura A, Kendoff D, Board TN. The current state of bearing surfaces in total hip replacement. Bone Joint J. 2014;96-B(2):147–56.
28. McKellop H, et al. Effect of sterilization method and other modifications on the wear resistance of acetabular cups made of ultra-high molecular weight polyethylene. A hip-simulator study. J Bone Joint Surg Am. 2000;82-A(12):1708–25.
29. Gordon AC, D'Lima DD, Colwell CW Jr. Highly cross-linked polyethylene in total hip arthroplasty. J Am Acad Orthop Surg. 2006;14(9):511–23.
30. Capello WN, et al. Continued improved wear with an annealed highly cross-linked polyethylene. Clin Orthop Relat Res. 2011;469(3):825–30.
31. Jacobs CA, et al. Clinical performance of highly cross-linked polyethylenes in total hip arthroplasty. J Bone Joint Surg Am. 2007;89(12):2779–86.
32. Bragdon CR, et al. The 2012 John Charnley Award: clinical multicenter studies of the wear performance of highly crosslinked remelted polyethylene in THA. Clin Orthop Relat Res. 2013;471(2):393–402.
33. Chatterji U, et al. Effect of total hip arthroplasty on recreational and sporting activity. ANZ J Surg. 2004;74(6):446–9.
34. Huch K, et al. Sports activities 5 years after total knee or hip arthroplasty: the Ulm Osteoarthritis Study. Ann Rheum Dis. 2005;64(12):1715–20.
35. Mallon WJ, Callaghan JJ. Total hip arthroplasty in active golfers. J Arthroplast. 1992;7(Suppl):339–46.
36. Williams DH, et al. Predictors of participation in sports after hip and knee arthroplasty. Clin Orthop Relat Res. 2012;470(2):555–61.

37. Wylde V, et al. Return to sport after joint replacement. J Bone Joint Surg Br. 2008;90(7):920–3.
38. Mont MA, et al. High-impact sports after total knee arthroplasty. J Arthroplast. 2008;23(6 Suppl 1):80–4.
39. Mont MA, et al. Tennis after total hip arthroplasty. Am J Sports Med. 1999;27(1):60–4.
40. van den Bogert AJ, Read L, Nigg BM. An analysis of hip joint loading during walking, running, and skiing. Med Sci Sports Exerc. 1999;31(1):131–42.
41. Gschwend N, et al. Alpine and cross-country skiing after total hip replacement: 2 cohorts of 50 patients each, one active, the other inactive in skiing, followed for 5-10 years. Acta Orthop Scand. 2000;71(3):243–9.
42. Lefevre N, et al. Return to judo after joint replacement. Knee Surg Sports Traumatol Arthrosc. 2013;21(12):2889–94.
43. Daniel J, et al. Blood and urine metal ion levels in young and active patients after Birmingham hip resurfacing arthroplasty: four-year results of a prospective longitudinal study. J Bone Joint Surg Br. 2007;89(2):169–73.
44. Pandit H, et al. Pseudotumours associated with metal-on-metal hip resurfacings. J Bone Joint Surg Br. 2008;90(7):847–51.
45. Klein GR, et al. Return to athletic activity after total hip arthroplasty. Consensus guidelines based on a survey of the Hip Society and American Association of Hip and Knee Surgeons. J Arthroplast. 2007;22(2):171–5.
46. Mancuso CA, et al. Randomized trials to modify patients' preoperative expectations of hip and knee arthroplasties. Clin Orthop Relat Res. 2008;466(2):424–31.
47. Bercik MJ, Joshi A, Parvizi J. Posterior cruciate-retaining versus posterior-stabilized total knee arthroplasty: a meta-analysis. J Arthroplasty. 2013;28(3):439–44.
48. Li N, et al. Posterior cruciate-retaining versus posterior stabilized total knee arthroplasty: a meta-analysis of randomized controlled trials. Knee Surg Sports Traumatol Arthrosc. 2014;22(3):556–64.
49. Jeffery RS, Morris RW, Denham RA. Coronal alignment after total knee replacement. J Bone Joint Surg Br. 1991;73(5):709–14.
50. D'Lima DD, et al. Polyethylene wear and variations in knee kinematics. Clin Orthop Relat Res. 2001;392:124–30.
51. Kuster MS, et al. Joint load considerations in total knee replacement. J Bone Joint Surg Br. 1997;79(1):109–13.
52. Kuster MS, et al. Endurance sports after total knee replacement: a biomechanical investigation. Med Sci Sports Exerc. 2000;32(4):721–4.
53. Kuster MS. Exercise recommendations after total joint replacement: a review of the current literature and proposal of scientifically based guidelines. Sports Med. 2002;32(7):433–45.
54. Chatterji U, et al. Effect of total knee arthroplasty on recreational and sporting activity. ANZ J Surg. 2005;75(6):405–8.
55. Bradbury N, et al. Participation in sports after total knee replacement. Am J Sports Med. 1998;26(4):530–5.
56. Dahm DL, et al. Patient-reported activity level after total knee arthroplasty. J Arthroplast. 2008;23(3):401–7.
57. Weiss JM, et al. What functional activities are important to patients with knee replacements? Clin Orthop Relat Res. 2002;404:172–88.
58. Hopper GP, Leach WJ. Participation in sporting activities following knee replacement: total versus unicompartmental. Knee Surg Sports Traumatol Arthrosc. 2008;16(10):973–9.
59. Mallon WJ, Callaghan JJ. Total knee arthroplasty in active golfers. J Arthroplast. 1993;8(3):299–306.
60. Hamai S, et al. Three-dimensional knee joint kinematics during golf swing and stationary cycling after total knee arthroplasty. J Orthop Res. 2008;26(12):1556–61.
61. D'Lima DD, et al. The Mark Coventry Award: in vivo knee forces during recreation and exercise after knee arthroplasty. Clin Orthop Relat Res. 2008;466(11):2605–11.

62. Healy WL, et al. Athletic activity after total joint arthroplasty. J Bone Joint Surg Am. 2008;90(10):2245–52.
63. Kozinn SC, Scott R. Unicondylar knee arthroplasty. J Bone Joint Surg Am. 1989;71(1):145–50.
64. Berend KR, Lombardi AV Jr. Liberal indications for minimally invasive oxford unicondylar arthroplasty provide rapid functional recovery and pain relief. Surg Technol Int. 2007;16:193–7.
65. Berger RA, et al. Results of unicompartmental knee arthroplasty at a minimum of ten years of follow-up. J Bone Joint Surg Am. 2005;87(5):999–1006.
66. Emerson RH Jr, Higgins LL. Unicompartmental knee arthroplasty with the oxford prosthesis in patients with medial compartment arthritis. J Bone Joint Surg Am. 2008;90(1):118–22.
67. Foran JR, et al. Long-term survivorship and failure modes of unicompartmental knee arthroplasty. Clin Orthop Relat Res. 2013;471(1):102–8.
68. Price AJ, Svard U. A second decade lifetable survival analysis of the Oxford unicompartmental knee arthroplasty. Clin Orthop Relat Res. 2011;469(1):174–9.
69. Lombardi AV Jr, et al. Is recovery faster for mobile-bearing unicompartmental than total knee arthroplasty? Clin Orthop Relat Res. 2009;467(6):1450–7.
70. Walton NP, et al. Patient-perceived outcomes and return to sport and work: TKA versus mini-incision unicompartmental knee arthroplasty. J Knee Surg. 2006;19(2):112–6.
71. Farr J, et al. Patellofemoral arthroplasty in the athlete. Clin Sports Med. 2014;33(3):547–52.

Chapter 15
Maximizing Performance and Preventing Injury in Masters Athletes

Christopher L. McCrum and Kellie K. Middleton

Age- and Sex-Related Changes in Athletic Performance

Masters athletes exhibit persistently high levels of functional capacity helping them advance through a healthy aging process. When evaluating the trend of top performances among masters athletes, performance continues to improve within age categories [1, 2]. However, the capacity for performance in athletics does decrease as people age. The rate of decline has been evaluated by several studies. When examining the track and field performance of senior athletes, both male and female performance decreased at approximately 3.4% for each year after the age of 50 in a relatively linear fashion, until the age of 75, where performance begins to fall more precipitously, with a decline of greater than 7% in performance times annually [3]. Furthermore, the age of maximum performance increases with greater race distances, and the rate of slowing as athletes age decreases as competition distances increase [4]. This is consistent with known shifts that take place within skeletal muscle: the percentages of slow-twitch type I muscle fibers increase with increasing age [5–11]. Similar findings are noted in other sports as well [12]. Masters swimmers also demonstrate a modest, linear decrease in performance of 0.6–1% per year until age 70, when a more rapid decline is noted [13, 14]. In Ironman triathletes, age-related rates of decline in performance are 13% for men and 15% for women each decade until age 70; with greater declines noted in swimming and running than cycling [1].

This pattern of an age-related decrease in performance is also noted in strength or power lifting athletes. Masters weightlifter performance deteriorates at approximately 1–1.5% per year, with a larger decrease in performance in the over 70 age

C. L. McCrum, MD (✉) · K. K. Middleton, MD, MPH
Department of Orthopaedic Surgery, University of Pittsburgh, Pittsburgh, PA, USA
e-mail: mccrumcl@upmc.edu; middletonkk@upmc.edu

© Springer International Publishing AG, part of Springer Nature 2018
V. J. Wright, K. K. Middleton (eds.), *Masterful Care of the Aging Athlete*,
https://doi.org/10.1007/978-3-319-16223-2_15

group [15]. It is noteworthy that the rate of decline in performance differs between endurance and anaerobic power athletes. Peak muscular power demonstrates a more rapid rate of decline with age than maximal aerobic capacity [16–19], which is evident when examining the rates of decline in performance in endurance versus peak power athletes, especially earlier in the aging process. Furthermore, the rate of decline of maximum voluntary force generation is greater for lower extremity muscles than upper extremity muscles [20], which suggests that athletes competing in different sports can show differing rates of decline in performance with aging.

Differences in performance decline are also noted between male and female master athletes. The performance of the female athlete decreases more rapidly over time compared to their male counterparts [3, 13]. This specific difference does appear to decrease over time. In masters swimmers, women were observed to be slower than men; however, they demonstrated a greater improvement in race times compared to men between ages 55 and 74. No difference existed in swimmers over the age of 80 [21, 22]. While the rate of decrease in performance does not differ in male masters athletes, performance data suggests that the decline in performance in sprinting is greater than that in endurance categories for female athletes, particularly in athletes greater than 75 years old [3].

In order to attain maximum performance with minimal injury risks, experts in exercise physiology and masters athlete training have advocated combining flexibility, aerobic intensity, resistance training, equilibrium and balance for a complete total body training regimen. Flexibility is improved through foam rolling and dynamic exercises during warm-ups, aerobic training with high-intensity workouts of shorter duration, and through resistance training with total body cross training. To increase flexibility, training focus is placed on equilibrium and balance. Such a routine helps master athletes achieve specific changes in musculoskeletal physiology in order to maximize performance through functional stretching, balanced muscle activity, and minimizing kinetic chain weaknesses. Increased intensity with less frequency allows the athlete to capitalize on the healthy aging process of cardiac and skeletal muscles' ability to maintain functional capacity while minimizing the burden of recovery that long workouts generally entail [23].

The Biology of Aging and Factors Affecting Performance

Muscle Function and Lean Muscle Mass

Muscular strength is decreased with aging, and this results in an impact on not only athletic activities but also the capacity of the elderly to accomplish activities of daily living [5, 6, 24–30]. The loss in strength is reflected by, and is proportional to, a decrease in muscle cross-sectional area [25]. Between the ages of 40 and 50 years, there can be a loss of 8% of muscle mass, and in the ensuing decades, this loss of muscle mass accelerates to more than 15% per decade after the age of 75 [24, 31].

Additionally, the decrease in muscle cross-sectional area observed in the elderly is also complicated by increases in fatty infiltration. While muscle power is mostly strictly related to cross-sectional area, high fat infiltration in muscle is associated with relatively decreased strength, muscle contractility, motor unit recruitment, and metabolism [32], as well as poorer performance with increased fat infiltration in muscle [33].

In addition to loss of frank muscle mass and fat infiltration of muscle, muscle composition changes with aging. Muscle is composed of both slow oxidative (slow-twitch type I) muscle and fast oxidative (fast-twitch type II) muscle. Slow oxidative fibers have a larger density of machinery for oxidative metabolism, including capillaries and mitochondria, as well as myoglobin, which contributes to the red color of healthy musculature. This muscle type is more efficient in aerobic, oxygen-consuming activities but is less efficient in performing high-power activities. Alternatively, fast oxidative muscle is rich in glycolytic enzymes and is characterized by fast, powerful contractions with poor endurance. With aging, there is a proportionally greater loss of the fast oxidative fibers compared with slow oxidative fibers [5–8]. This loss of type II muscle fibers is primarily associated with a loss of the number of muscle fibers, as well as a decrease in fiber size [34].

The implication on such age-related changes on masters athletes is less clear. Some authors have suggested that masters runners and swimmers have similar muscle fiber composition to that of age-matched controls [6], though others have found that masters athletes' muscle fiber composition profiles matched those of similarly trained younger athletes [5].

Endurance Capacity

Cardiovascular age-related changes begin early in life with maximal heart rate (HRmax) decreasing 1 beat per year (or 10 beats/min per decade) beginning at age 10. Notably, these declines do not reflect exercise status [35–37]. Although cardiovascular function is known to decrease with aging, masters athletes can continue competing at a high level of endurance through adaptations consistent with those of younger athletes.

Maximal oxygen consumption (VO_2max) is the maximum volume of oxygen available in circulation to produce energy within cells via oxidative pathways. A change in VO_2max is one of the key metrics in maximizing performance in masters athletes. Although decreases in maximal cardiac output, stroke volume (or the amount of blood sent into circulation with each heartbeat), and maximal heart rate all contribute to decreased aerobic capacity [38], given that the maximal heart rate shows minimal response to training, the primary method an athlete can increase his or her VO_2max is through physiologic changes to the cardiovascular system that increase stroke volume.

In sedentary adults, the VO_2max decreases 10% per decade after the age of 25. With training, this decrease can be halved in masters athletes [37, 39]. Trappe et al.

found in their masters level runners a 5.2% decrease in absolute VO_2max and 13.4% decrease in their relative VO_2max over a 22-year period. The initial average age was 25.7 years, and the follow-up average age was 47.2 years [39]. The decrease in observed VO_2max averages to a 6% loss per decade, which is consistent with results elsewhere in the literature [40]. Similar studies in athletes between 45 and 65 years old noted a total 12% decrease over 20 years, with only a 3% change observed until the seventh decade of life. The authors attribute the ability to maintain VO_2max while aging to following a consistent training regimen, remaining at optimal body-weight, having normal resting blood pressure and peripheral vascular resistance, maintaining relatively high energy output, and having an above average cardiac reserve [37]. Cardiac adaptations in older endurance athletes are most pronounced by left ventricular hypertrophy, resulting in improved systolic performance during peak exercise, which in turn, leads to enhanced stroke volume [41]. Evidence suggests that there may be an acceleration in VO_2max losses during the sixth decade, but a decrease in training frequency likely contributes to this rapid change [37, 42, 43].

The capacity for the lungs to facilitate oxygen diffusion into the blood is also affected by age. Lung capacity declines approximately 250 mL per decade. Additionally, between the ages of 20 and 70, maximum lung capacity declines by 40%. This is related to changes in tissue quality and composition resulting in decreased lung tissue elasticity, decreased capillary density, and diminished quality of oxygen perfusion across membranes [23].

Lactate threshold is higher in masters athletes compared to that of younger athletes [5]. The lactate threshold is the point where oxidative processes are unable to meet the demand for oxygen production, and anaerobic processes are engaged to produce energy resulting in the production of lactic acid as a by-product [23]. Given that VO_2max declines with age, the rate at which the lactate threshold is reached is different in masters athlete compared to younger, similarly trained athletes. Fortunately, physiologic changes can occur in highly trained masters athletes to help compensate for this difference. The muscle of masters athletes have a higher level of succinate dehydrogenase and β-hydroxyacyl-CoA dehydrogenase activity and lower lactate dehydrogenase activity than younger athletes. This difference in enzymatic activity allows masters athletes to compensate for a decreased VO_2max [5].

Training Intensity

Training intensity is a critical consideration when considering both the capacity for performance and the risk of injury in the masters athlete. Athletes tend to train and compete less frequently as they age [43, 44]. As a result, athletes have fewer opportunities to improve frequency-driven performance measures, such as VO_2max, muscular strength and endurance, and exercise economy [23].

Masters athlete performance following short recovery periods is also decreased compared with their younger counterparts. When examining cycling performance after 10, 24, and 48 h after training, masters athletes demonstrate poorer performance as well as lower rates of muscle protein repair and remodeling [45].

Following muscle-damaging exercise, masters athletes experience slower recovery rates compared with similarly trained younger athletes. Given that these differences are not noted in non-muscle-damaging exercise, it appears that this difference is related to decreased protein remodeling in the masters athlete. Diet may play a greater role in recovery following exercise-induced muscle damage in the masters athlete [46].

Sport Mechanics and Exercise Economy

Sport-specific fluidity and locomotion can be altered with physiologic, age-related changes. For instance, aging sprinters have markedly shorter strides than training matched younger runners, as a result of decreased muscle power and joint flexibility [23]. This occurs as connective tissues in muscle and tendons have increased stiffness in age, resulting in a decrease in joint range of motion. In the knee, up to 33% of range of motion can be lost in the masters athlete. This leads to the stride transition occurring near an athlete's maximal knee flexion, which decreases one's ability to use the power generated for the next stride [47].

Sport-specific mechanics are important to consider when evaluating performance changes in the aging athlete. Since power decreases at a more rapid rate than endurance capacity, athletes engaged in sports that require greater amounts of power are more likely to experience an increased rate of decline in performance with age. For instance, the power output in running is linearly related to velocity, while the mechanical advantage of a bicycle makes the power output dependent on the velocity to the third power. This results in slower decline in cycling performance compared with sprinting performance as an athlete ages [2].

Sports-Related Injuries and Medical Issues Impacting Masters Athletes

Sports-Related Injuries and Injury Prevention

The masters athlete is more likely to experience sports-related injuries as tendons, ligaments, cartilage, and muscle in those of advanced age are more susceptible to trauma. Furthermore, such injuries heal with greater difficulty than those of younger, similarly trained athletes [49]. Injuries of the lower extremity are more frequent than those in other areas of the body, with sprains being the most common injury and the knee being the most frequently affected joint [49, 50]. Meniscal tears, Achilles tendinopathies, and rotator cuff injuries are among the most common injuries affecting masters athletes [51].

Masters athletes are susceptible to suffering both acute traumatic injuries and chronic injuries associated with overuse. Since the aging body has a diminished ability to adapt to high levels of training, there is a resulting decrease in the safety margin to the dose of exercise [49]. However, the incidence of inflammatory overuse injuries is greater than acute injuries, with 70–85% of masters athletes injuries falling within this category [3, 52]. Furthermore, injuries are simply common in older athletes, with a reported incidence up to over 80% [50]. Unfortunately, sports-related injuries sustained by masters athletes can persist for more than 1 year after onset [53].

Before exercise, warming up not only functions to raise one's body temperature, it also helps prepare the musculoskeletal system for exertion. As such, it is essential to an athlete's training and should not be neglected. A good pre-training warm-up should be dynamic and sport-specific in an effort to help increase exercise economy and reduce the risk of injury. An effective warm-up will increase blood flow to sport-relevant muscle groups, allow for efficient contraction and relaxation of both agonist and antagonism muscles, decrease the resistance to motion of tendon and muscle, and facilitate oxygen delivery to tissues by increasing temperature and circulation. Dynamic warm-ups allow muscle lengthening and contraction, which provides a more functional range of motion than traditional static stretching. Stretching can still be appropriately employed following exercise. Dynamic warm-ups further contribute to exercise performance by preparing the body to mobilize in specific sport-specific movement patterns [23].

Another factor that may be more unique to the population of masters athletes is the impact of certain medications on the body and how they affect the cardiovascular and/or musculoskeletal systems. For instance, many older individuals are on medications in the statin family to help lower circulating cholesterol. Statins have a well-known side effect of myalgia and increased fatigability; however, Terpak et al. found that these medications do not cause enough fatigue or pain in masters swimmers to require a decrease in duration or intensity of workouts [54]. Additionally, while some evidence suggests that coenzyme Q10 (CoQ10) supplementation of 50 mg twice daily can reduce statin-related muscular symptoms [55], there is increasing evidence to the contrary [56, 57]. In essence, both physicians and masters athletes alike should simply be aware of medication side effect profiles and their potential impact on training.

Cardiovascular Disease and Exercise Precautions

While musculoskeletal injuries can be commonplace in the masters athletes, consensus recommendations call for a formal pre-participation evaluation of the masters athletes. A pre-participation history and physical is particularly important to identify any cardiovascular issues. Potentially catastrophic events can result from missed conditions [58]: exercise-related myocardial infarction is not uncommon in the older athlete population [59–63]. When examining masters athletes, it is important to gather information with respect to the athlete's overall health including other age-relevant parameters such as vision loss, diabetes, and hypertension.

Medical evaluation should begin with the American Heart Association pre-participation screening history including a family history of premature sudden cardiac death or heart disease in surviving relatives, as well as personal history for heart murmur, systemic hypertension, fatigability, syncope, and exertional dyspnea [64]. Standard 12-lead electrocardiogram (ECG) has limited diagnostic value in the masters athlete; however, it can detect less common conditions in the population such as hypertrophic cardiomyopathy and arrhythmias. An exercise ECG should be considered for any patient with moderate to high risk for coronary artery disease before participation. Specific subgroups that should be considered include men over 40–45 years old and women over 50–55 years old, individuals diagnosed with hypercholesterolemia/dyslipidemia or systemic hypertension, and individuals with a history of recent or current cigarette smoking, diabetes mellitus, myocardial infarction, sudden cardiac death in a first-degree relative less than 60 years old, an individual with any symptoms suggestive of underlying coronary artery disease, or any athlete 65 years or older *without* the aforementioned risk factors [58].

Not only should masters athletes undergo a pre-participation physical, they should regularly follow-up with their primary care physician to ensure their optimal health while training. To promote overall athlete health and ensure safe training, additional recommendations encourage that blood pressure be normalized before training or competition. Although mild hypertension should not restrict competitive masters athletes sports eligibility, athletes with moderate (>160 mmHg systolic or 110 mmHg diastolic) hypertension should be restricted until blood pressure control is achieved. Furthermore, these athletes should continue to be followed at least every 2 months to monitor control [65].

Utmost care should be taken with regard to disqualifying athletes from high-intensity activities, should there be sufficient concern for potential catastrophic events. Occasionally, some masters athletes are not cleared for a particular competition or certain training exercises. Discerning which activities and/or competitions should be restricted is especially important given that the physiologic impact of competitive events may mask crucial warning signs precipitating a major health event. Specific recommendations exist restricting high-intensity competitive sports for patients with impaired left ventricular systolic function less than 50% in resting conditions, evidence of exercise-induced ischemia including angina or positive ECG, evidence of exercise-induced arrhythmias, and exercise-induced systolic hypotension [58]. Dilated cardiomyopathy warrants activity restriction, and patients with evidence or history of endocarditis should be held from activity for at least 6 months after their symptoms have resolved [64].

The Impact of Osteoarthritis and Exercise Precautions

Running is a high-impact activity and can have deleterious effects on lower extremity joint health in masters athletes. In fact, controversy exists on whether or not running increases the rate of (or progression of) osteoarthritis (OA) in knees and hips. There has been an increased association noted between elite participation in weight-bearing sports and radiographic evidence of osteoarthritis, but the overall impact with regard to arthroplasty and athletic performance is unclear and appears more closely related to single-impact insults and repetitive microtrauma as opposed to regular intense activity [66]. While several studies have suggested that running increases the risk and progression of knee osteoarthritis [67, 68], others have refuted such a link [69, 70]. The overall quality of evidence is lacking. While osteoarthritis is not a contraindication to general exercise, certain modifications should be recommended in order to optimize athlete performance and minimize the contribution of exercise to the progression of degenerative joint disease [66, 71]. The Cochrane review of patients with knee OA evaluated the impact of exercise on patient's disease. From this review, simple quadriceps strengthening is recommended to help decrease knee pain [71]. In general, an effort should be made to minimize impacting forces through lower extremity joints, with strategies such as avoidance of running on hard surfaces (e.g., asphalt and treadmills), weight loss, quadriceps strengthening, and choosing well-padded supportive shoe wear that is replaced at appropriate intervals.

Conclusion

Along with decreased age-related declines in cardiovascular function, muscle strength, endurance capacity, and recovery from changes, masters athletes also show improved neuromuscular stability compared with aged-matched sedentary controls [48]. Regardless of the known benefits of exercise in aging populations, care must be taken to ensure that an athlete's musculoskeletal and cardiovascular systems are capable of withstanding the physiological stress of training. Only then can the benefits of exercise be truly realized and fully appreciated by masters athletes.

References

1. Bernard T, Sultana F, Lepers R, Hausswirth C, Brisswalter J. Age-related decline in olympic triathlon performance: effect of locomotion mode. Exp Aging Res. 2010;36(1):64–78.
2. Lepers R, Rüst CA, Stapley PJ, Knechtle B. Relative improvements in endurance performance with age: evidence from 25 years of Hawaii Ironman racing. Age (Dordr). 2013;35(3):953–62.
3. Wright VJ, Perricelli BC. Age-related rates of decline in performance among elite senior athletes. Am J Sports Med. 2008;36(3):443–50.
4. Moore DH. A study of age group track and field records to relate age and running speed. Nature. 1975;253(5489):264–5.
5. Coggan AR, Spina RJ, Rogers MA, et al. Histochemical and enzymatic characteristics of skeletal muscle in master athletes. J Appl Physiol (1985). 1990;68(5):1896–901.
6. Klitgaard H, Mantoni M, Schiaffino S, et al. Function, morphology and protein expression of ageing skeletal muscle: a cross-sectional study of elderly men with different training backgrounds. Acta Physiol Scand. 1990;140(1):41–54.

7. Grimby G, Danneskiold-Samsøe B, Hvid K, Saltin B. Morphology and enzymatic capacity in arm and leg muscles in 78-81 year old men and women. Acta Physiol Scand. 1982;115(1):125–34.
8. Lexell J, Taylor CC, Sjöström M. What is the cause of the ageing atrophy? Total number, size and proportion of different fiber types studied in whole vastus lateralis muscle from 15- to 83-year-old men. J Neurol Sci. 1988;84(2–3):275–94.
9. Klitgaard H, Zhou M, Schiaffino S, Betto R, Salviati G, Saltin B. Ageing alters the myosin heavy chain composition of single fibres from human skeletal muscle. Acta Physiol Scand. 1990;140(1):55–62.
10. Orlander J, Aniansson A. Effect of physical training on skeletal muscle metabolism and ultrastructure in 70 to 75-year-old men. Acta Physiol Scand. 1980;109(2):149–54.
11. Lexell J, Downham DY. The occurrence of fibre-type grouping in healthy human muscle: a quantitative study of cross-sections of whole vastus lateralis from men between 15 and 83 years. Acta Neuropathol (Berl). 1991;81(4):377–81.
12. Baker AB, Tang YQ. Aging performance for masters records in athletics, swimming, rowing, cycling, triathlon, and weightlifting. Exp Aging Res. 2010;36(4):453–77.
13. Donato AJ, Tench K, Glueck DH, Seals DR, Eskurza I, Tanaka H. Declines in physiological functional capacity with age: a longitudinal study in peak swimming performance. J Appl Physiol (1985). 2003;94(2):764–9.
14. Rubin RT, Rahe RH. Effects of aging in Masters swimmers: 40-year review and suggestions for optimal health benefits. Open Access J Sports Med. 2010;1:39–44.
15. Meltzer DE. Age dependence of Olympic weightlifting ability. Med Sci Sports Exerc. 1994;26(8):1053–67.
16. Buskirk ER, Hodgson JL. Age and aerobic power: the rate of change in men and women. Fed Proc. 1987;46(5):1824–9.
17. Grimby G, Saltin B. The ageing muscle. Clin Physiol. 1983;3(3):209–18.
18. Larsson L, Grimby G, Karlsson J. Muscle strength and speed of movement in relation to age and muscle morphology. J Appl Physiol. 1979;46(3):451–6.
19. Bortz WM, Bortz WM. How fast do we age? Exercise performance over time as a biomarker. J Gerontol A Biol Sci Med Sci. 1996;51(5):M223–5.
20. McDonagh MJ, White MJ, Davies CT. Different effects of ageing on the mechanical properties of human arm and leg muscles. Gerontology. 1984;30(1):49–54.
21. Knechtle B, Nikolaidis PT, König S, Rosemann T, Rüst CA. Performance trends in master freestyle swimmers aged 25-89 years at the FINA World Championships from 1986 to 2014. Age (Dordr). 2016;38(1):18.
22. Unterweger CM, Knechtle B, Nikolaidis PT, Rosemann T, Rüst CA. Increased participation and improved performance in age group backstroke master swimmers from 25-29 to 100-104 years at the FINA World Masters Championships from 1986 to 2014. SpringerPlus. 2016;5:645.
23. Wright VJ. Masterful care of the aging triathlete. Sports Med Arthrosc Rev. 2012;20(4):231–6.
24. Fiatarone MA, Marks EC, Ryan ND, Meredith CN, Lipsitz LA, Evans WJ. High-intensity strength training in nonagenarians. Effects on skeletal muscle. JAMA. 1990;263(22):3029–34.
25. Frontera WR, Hughes VA, Lutz KJ, Evans WJ. A cross-sectional study of muscle strength and mass in 45- to 78-yr-old men and women. J Appl Physiol (1985). 1991;71(2):644–50.
26. Bassey EJ, Fiatarone MA, O'Neill EF, Kelly M, Evans WJ, Lipsitz LA. Leg extensor power and functional performance in very old men and women. Clin Sci (Lond). 1992;82(3):321–7.
27. Aniansson A, Sperling L, Rundgren A, Lehnberg E. Muscle function in 75-year-old men and women. A longitudinal study. Scand J Rehabil Med Suppl. 1983;9:92–102.
28. Davies CT, Thomas DO, White MJ. Mechanical properties of young and elderly human muscle. Acta Med Scand Suppl. 1986;711:219–26.
29. Fiatarone MA, O'Neill EF, Ryan ND, et al. Exercise training and nutritional supplementation for physical frailty in very elderly people. N Engl J Med. 1994;330(25):1769–75.
30. Young A, Stokes M, Crowe M. The size and strength of the quadriceps muscles of old and young men. Clin Physiol. 1985;5(2):145–54.

31. Evans SL, Davy KP, Stevenson ET, Seals DR. Physiological determinants of 10-km performance in highly trained female runners of different ages. J Appl Physiol (1985). 1995;78(5):1931–41.
32. Baumgartner RN, Koehler KM, Gallagher D, et al. Epidemiology of sarcopenia among the elderly in New Mexico. Am J Epidemiol. 1998;147(8):755–63.
33. Visser M, Kritchevsky SB, Goodpaster BH, et al. Leg muscle mass and composition in relation to lower extremity performance in men and women aged 70 to 79: the health, aging and body composition study. J Am Geriatr Soc. 2002;50(5):897–904.
34. Brunner F, Schmid A, Sheikhzadeh A, Nordin M, Yoon J, Frankel V. Effects of aging on Type II muscle fibers: a systematic review of the literature. J Aging Phys Act. 2007;15(3):336–48.
35. Fitzgerald MD, Tanaka H, Tran ZV, Seals DR. Age-related declines in maximal aerobic capacity in regularly exercising vs. sedentary women: a meta-analysis. J Appl Physiol (1985). 1997;83(1):160–5.
36. Eskurza I, Donato AJ, Moreau KL, Seals DR, Tanaka H. Changes in maximal aerobic capacity with age in endurance-trained women: 7-yr follow-up. J Appl Physiol (1985). 2002;92(6):2303–8.
37. Kasch FW, Wallace JP, Van Camp SP, Verity L. A longitudinal study of cardiovascular stability in active men aged 45 to 65 years. Phys Sportsmed. 1988;16(1):117–24.
38. Ogawa T, Spina RJ, Martin WH, et al. Effects of aging, sex, and physical training on cardiovascular responses to exercise. Circulation. 1992;86(2):494–503.
39. Trappe SW, Costill DL, Vukovich MD, Jones J, Melham T. Aging among elite distance runners: a 22-yr longitudinal study. J Appl Physiol (1985). 1996;80(1):285–90.
40. Rogers MA, Hagberg JM, Martin WH, Ehsani AA, Holloszy JO. Decline in VO2max with aging in master athletes and sedentary men. J Appl Physiol (1985). 1990;68(5):2195–9.
41. Seals DR, Hagberg JM, Spina RJ, Rogers MA, Schechtman KB, Ehsani AA. Enhanced left ventricular performance in endurance trained older men. Circulation. 1994;89(1):198–205.
42. Pollock ML, Mengelkoch LJ, Graves JE, et al. Twenty-year follow-up of aerobic power and body composition of older track athletes. J Appl Physiol (1985). 1997;82(5):1508–16.
43. Maharam LG, Bauman PA, Kalman D, Skolnik H, Perle SM. Masters athletes: factors affecting performance. Sports Med. 1999;28(4):273–85.
44. Medic N, Starkes JL, Young BW. Examining relative age effects on performance achievement and participation rates in Masters athletes. J Sports Sci. 2007;25(12):1377–84.
45. Doering TM, Jenkins DG, Reaburn PR, Borges NR, Hohmann E, Phillips SM. Lower integrated muscle protein synthesis in masters compared with younger athletes. Med Sci Sports Exerc. 2016;48(8):1613–8.
46. Doering TM, Reaburn PR, Phillips SM, Jenkins DG. Postexercise dietary protein strategies to maximize skeletal muscle repair and remodeling in masters endurance athletes: a review. Int J Sport Nutr Exerc Metab. 2016;26(2):168–78.
47. Troop B. Training for masters athletes. London: UK Peak Performance Publishing; 2004.
48. Power GA, Allen MD, Gilmore KJ, et al. Motor unit number and transmission stability in octogenarian world class athletes: can age-related deficits be outrun? J Appl Physiol (1985). 2016;121(4):1013–20.
49. Kallinen M, Markku A. Aging, physical activity and sports injuries. An overview of common sports injuries in the elderly. Sports Med. 1995;20(1):41–52.
50. Kallinen M, Alén M. Sports-related injuries in elderly men still active in sports. Br J Sports Med. 1994;28(1):52–5.
51. Galloway MT, Jokl P. Aging successfully: the importance of physical activity in maintaining health and function. J Am Acad Orthop Surg. 2000;8(1):37–44.
52. Kannus P, Niittymäki S, Järvinen M, Lehto M. Sports injuries in elderly athletes: a three-year prospective, controlled study. Age Ageing. 1989;18(4):263–70.
53. Tayrose GA, Beutel BG, Cardone DA, Sherman OH. The masters athlete. Sports Health. 2015;7(3):270–6.
54. Terpak K, Guthrie S, Erickson S. Statin use and self-reported swimming performance in US masters swimmers. J Sports Sci. 2015;33(3):286–92.

55. Skarlovnik A, Janić M, Lunder M, Turk M, Šabovič M. Coenzyme Q10 supplementation decreases statin-related mild-to-moderate muscle symptoms: a randomized clinical study. Med Sci Monit. 2014;20:2183–8.
56. Taylor BA, Lorson L, White CM, Thompson PD. A randomized trial of coenzyme Q10 in patients with confirmed statin myopathy. Atherosclerosis. 2015;238(2):329–35.
57. Schaars CF, Stalenhoef AFH. Effects of ubiquinone (coenzyme Q10) on myopathy in statin users. Curr Opin Lipidol. 2008;19(6):553–7.
58. Maron BJ, Araújo CG, Thompson PD, et al. Recommendations for preparticipation screening and the assessment of cardiovascular disease in masters athletes: an advisory for healthcare professionals from the working groups of the World Heart Federation, the International Federation of Sports Medicine, and the American Heart Association Committee on Exercise, Cardiac Rehabilitation, and Prevention. Circulation. 2001;103(2):327–34.
59. Mittleman MA, Maclure M, Tofler GH, Sherwood JB, Goldberg RJ, Muller JE. Triggering of acute myocardial infarction by heavy physical exertion. Protection against triggering by regular exertion. Determinants of Myocardial Infarction Onset Study Investigators. N Engl J Med. 1993;329(23):1677–83.
60. Willich SN, Lewis M, Löwel H, Arntz HR, Schubert F, Schröder R. Physical exertion as a trigger of acute myocardial infarction. Triggers and Mechanisms of Myocardial Infarction Study Group. N Engl J Med. 1993;329(23):1684–90.
61. Gibbons LW, Cooper KH, Meyer BM, Ellison RC. The acute cardiac risk of strenuous exercise. JAMA. 1980;244(16):1799–801.
62. Rich MW. Risk for sudden cardiac death associated with marathon running. J Am Coll Cardiol. 1997;29(1):224.
63. Waller BF, Roberts WC. Sudden death while running in conditioned runners aged 40 years or over. Am J Cardiol. 1980;45(6):1292–300.
64. Maron BJ, Thompson PD, Puffer JC, et al. Cardiovascular preparticipation screening of competitive athletes: addendum: an addendum to a statement for health professionals from the Sudden Death Committee (Council on Clinical Cardiology) and the Congenital Cardiac Defects Committee (Council on Cardiovascular Disease in the Young), American Heart Association. Circulation. 1998;97(22):2294.
65. Thompson PD, Klocke FJ, Levine BD, Van Camp SP. 26th Bethesda conference: recommendations for determining eligibility for competition in athletes with cardiovascular abnormalities. Task Force 5: coronary artery disease. Med Sci Sports Exerc. 1994;26(10 Suppl):S271–5.
66. Wolf BR, Amendola A. Impact of osteoarthritis on sports careers. Clin Sports Med. 2005;24(1):187–98.
67. Felson DT, Niu J, Clancy M, Sack B, Aliabadi P, Zhang Y. Effect of recreational physical activities on the development of knee osteoarthritis in older adults of different weights: the Framingham Study. Arthritis Rheum. 2007;57(1):6–12.
68. Kujala UM, Sarna S, Kaprio J, Koskenvuo M, Karjalainen J. Heart attacks and lower-limb function in master endurance athletes. Med Sci Sports Exerc. 1999;31(7):1041–6.
69. Richmond SA, Fukuchi RK, Ezzat A, Schneider K, Schneider G, Emery CA. Are joint injury, sport activity, physical activity, obesity, or occupational activities predictors for osteoarthritis? A systematic review. J Orthop Sports Phys Ther. 2013;43(8):515–B19.
70. Timmins KA, Leech RD, Batt ME, Edwards KL. Running and Knee osteoarthritis: a systematic review and meta-analysis. Am J Sports Med. 2017;45(6):1447–57.
71. Fransen M, McConnell S, Hernandez-Molina G, Reichenbach S. Exercise for osteoarthritis of the hip. Cochrane Database Syst Rev. 2009;3:CD007912.

Chapter 16
An Exercise Prescription for Healthy Active Aging

Dukens LaBaze, Jared Anthony Crasto, and Kellie K. Middleton

Abbreviations

AM	Attentional matrices
AT	Aerobic training
CDC	Centers for Disease Control and Prevention
DBP	Diastolic blood pressure
ERFC	French rapid evaluation of cognitive function
HDL	High-density lipoprotein
LDL	Low-density lipoprotein
MAP	Mean arterial pressure
MMSE	Mini-mental status examination
NCOA	National Council on Aging
PAGs	Physical activity guidelines
SBP	Systolic blood pressure
SF-36	Short Form Health Survey
T2DM	Type 2 diabetes mellitus
TC	Total cholesterol
TMT	Trail making test
VLMT	Verbal learning and memory test
WHO	World Health Organization

D. LaBaze, BS · J. A. Crasto, MD (✉) · K. K. Middleton, MD, MPH
Department of Orthopaedic Surgery, University of Pittsburgh Medical Center,
Pittsburgh, PA, USA
e-mail: CrastoJA@upmc.edu; middletonkk@upmc.edu

© Springer International Publishing AG, part of Springer Nature 2018
V. J. Wright, K. K. Middleton (eds.), *Masterful Care of the Aging Athlete*,
https://doi.org/10.1007/978-3-319-16223-2_16

Background

Physical inactivity has been described as the fourth leading risk factor contributing to deaths and burden of disease globally—ranking higher than obesity [1]. Chronic diseases such as diabetes mellitus type II, hypertension, hypercholesterolemia, obesity, and osteoporosis (which can lead to fragility fractures) are a major cause of physical, psychological, and social morbidity and mortality in the United States. Any effort to promote healthy aging and prevention can significantly decrease the burden of chronic disease. In this chapter, the musculoskeletal impact of physical activity will be discussed as the physiologic cardiovascular and metabolic benefits of exercise are outside the scope of this textbook.

As our growing population ages, there becomes increasing pressure on the healthcare systems and services that serve it. The World Health Organization (WHO) estimates that by the year 2050, the number of adults aged 65 or older will double [2]. As life expectancy is increasing, by the year 2050 the global number of adults aged 80 or older will be about 268 million in less-developed countries and 124 million in developed countries [3]. The dramatic increase in this age group generates an imperative need for preventive medicine. While many factors may play a role in the healthy aging process, exercise has been demonstrated to benefit a myriad of processes in the aging individual [4–6].

In patients older than 65 years, physical activity preserves muscle mass and strength, which assist in slowing the age-related regression in functional capacity [7]. The National Council on Aging (NCOA) reports there are 27,000 deaths per year related to elderly falls [8]. Community-based trials demonstrate as high as a 32% decrease in fall risk with a 66% reduction in fall-related fractures in older individuals who regularly exercise [9, 10]. Quality of life—assessed with MacNew or Short Form Health Survey score (SF-36)—increased 178% simply with exercise [11].

Benefits of Exercise

There are many benefits of exercise for the aging population [4, 12]. No matter how sedentary and individual is at the present moment, he or she can incrementally modify risks factors for chronic disease by starting and continuing to engage in physical activity. Benefits include chronic disease prevention and risk reduction, functional status benefits, psychological well-being, and social benefits [4] (Fig. 16.1). The Centers for Disease Control and Prevention (CDC) reports that every 4 min one American dies from a stroke [13]. Physical activity has been demonstrated to lower the risk of stroke across various age groups and populations [14, 15]. Moderate and vigorous physical activity decrease the relative risk of developing a stroke up to 15% and 22%, respectively. Though the mechanism is controversial, physical activity improves cognitive function, reduces occurrence of dementia, and improves the health of patients who have dementia [16–18]. Inactivity is the most significant risk

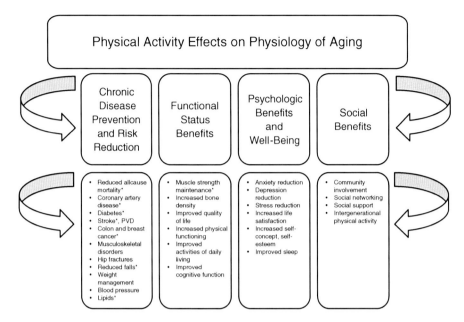

Fig. 16.1 Framework for the potential benefits of physical activity in older adults. (Asterkisk) Denotes "strong" epidemiological evidence as described by the US Department of Health and Human Services' 2008 Physical Activity Guidelines Advisory Report. (http://www.health.gov/paguidelines/guidelines)

factor for developing Alzheimer's dementia. In physically active older patients, the risk of developing dementia is reduced by 28% [17, 19]. Mental health is also positively impacted by exercise, with symptoms of anxiety and depression are reduced with physical activity [20–23].

Maintaining functional status with aging is important for preserving quality of life, reduced fall risk, and decreased healthcare costs [24, 25]. *Overall Benefits:* Recent systematic reviews focusing on seniors demonstrated consistent evidence that aerobic training yields benefits on cardiopulmonary fitness, hypertension, glucose metabolism, functional outcomes (such as muscle strength, physical performance, risk of falling), cognitive performance, and quality of life [5, 26–29]. *Cardiopulmonary (peak exercise capacity):* Aerobic training has a profound effect on cardiopulmonary fitness, in particular. It increases peak exercise capacity, which is an important predictor of mortality over other established risk factors for cardiovascular disease [5]. In a study examining over 6000 men referred for treadmill exercise stress testing for a clinical reason, predictors of mortality included older age, lower maximal heart rates, lower maximal systolic and diastolic blood pressures, and lower exercise capacity [30]. In this study, peak exercise capacity became a strong predictor of the risk of death among both healthy subjects and those with cardiovascular disease. *Cognition:* Exercise has also demonstrated measureable improvements in cognition. A recent large review demonstrated

4–34% cognitive improvement as measured on multiple cognitive function tests including the mini-mental status examination (MMSE), verbal learning and memory test (VLMT), French Rapid Evaluation of Cognitive Function (ERFC) test, Trail Making Test (TMT), attentional matrices (AM) test, and Wisconsin card-sorting test [5].

Aerobic training in the advanced age populations has been shown to exert a positive influence on blood pressure in both healthy seniors *and* obese seniors with mild to moderate hypertension (treated or untreated) and type 2 diabetes mellitus. Aerobic training has been shown to decrease systolic blood pressure (SBP), diastolic blood pressure (DBP), and mean arterial pressure (MAP) up to 16%, 13%, and 11.5%, respectively [31–37]. However, elderly with severe but treated hypertension had no change in SBP and DBP with AT [38]. Type 2 diabetes mellitus (T2DM) is another preventable disease shown to improve with exercise. Elderly patients who are healthy or have T2DM managed with oral anti-diabetic medications have demonstrated tighter glycemic control when evaluated by hemoglobin A1C, oral glucose tolerance, fasting insulin, fasting glucose, insulin sensitivity index, and glucose disposal rate [39–44]. Hyperlipidemia is a well-established risk factor for atherosclerosis and is common in elderly patients. AT decreases triglycerides, total cholesterol (TC), low-density lipoprotein (LDL), high-density lipoprotein (HDL), and TC/HDL ratio; positive outcomes have also been observed in patients with multiple comorbidities [43, 44].

Physical Activity Guidelines

In 2010, the WHO released physical activity guidelines (PAGs), comprising specific recommendations for strength and balance or flexibility, as well as for aerobic (large muscle) activity throughout a typical week [45]. The overall total volume of physical activity should include 150 min per week of moderate-intensity aerobic physical activity or 75 min per week of vigorous-intensity aerobic physical activity, with the upper limits of 300 and 150 min, respectively. Additionally, balance training should be performed three or more days per week and muscle strengthening 2 or more days per week for fall prevention [45] (Fig. 16.2).

Special considerations have been made for those who are considered "frail." Individuals who meet three of the following five phenotypic criteria indicating compromised function are considered frail: low grip strength, low energy, slowed walking speed, low physical activity level, unintentional weight loss [46]. In these groups, guidelines suggest more focus on muscle strengthening via resistance training. Resistance training has demonstrated excellent outcomes in the frail population in specific [47]. Resistance training is postulated to enhance aerobic capacity and subsequently result in an increased ability to engage in endurance activities such as walking and also in balance training to provide maximal benefit. Thus, resistance training is key in enabling other forms of beneficial exercise specifically in the "frail" population.

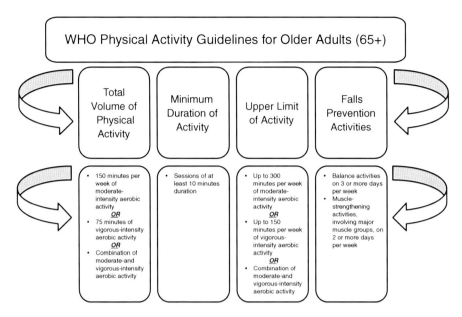

Fig. 16.2 World Health Organization Physical Activity Guidelines for Older Adults (65 years and older)

Elderly Individual Perspectives

Physical inactivity is responsible for as many as 9% of deaths worldwide and among the top 10 risk factors for global risk burden; however 30% of the world's population still fails to reach adequate levels of physical activity [1, 48, 49]. A recent large-scale review of 132 studies, encompassing almost 6000 participants, was conducted to examine the perspectives of elderly individuals in regard to exercise for the aging population [6].

Positive social influences included valuing interaction with peers and encouragement from others. Sixty-four percent of studies demonstrated that participants valued social contact; enjoyed seeing familiar faces when exercising, and/or preferred group-based activities because they developed a sense of belonging, enjoyment, and establishment of friendships. Sixty-two percent of studies demonstrated that encouragement from others was essential. This included verbal encouragement, practical help (such as transportation), or purchased equipment (such as a pedometer or bike) provided by friends and family. Negative social influences included dependence on professional instruction and social awkwardness. Thirty percent of studies demonstrated that participants believed the presence or quality of exercise instructors influenced their exercise behavior—and even that exercising without instructors was potentially unsafe. Twenty-two percent of studies demonstrated that participants experienced a lack of confidence in social settings, apprehension about meeting others, and pressure to keep pace with the class—leading to a sense of incompetence and decreased likelihood to continue exercising [6].

Perceptions of physical limitations also prevented participants from continuing exercise. Fifty-six percent of studies indicated that symptoms and physical limitations caused by existing comorbidities prevented participants from exercising. Forty percent of studies showed that competing priorities (such as caring for family or work responsibilities) prohibited participants from exercising. Thirty-four percent of studies found that pain or discomfort caused by the exercise was a deterrent. Twenty-eight percent of studies found participant concerns about falling for fear of injury (especially if previous injury was sustained from a fall) was a deterrent. Access difficulties such as poor transportation, unsuitable weather, unavailability of programs, and affordability were also deterrents [6].

Interestingly, the perceived benefits of physical activity were mixed. Only in 52% of studies did participants believe that exercise would enhance their strength, balance, and flexibility. In 20% of studies, participants believed exercise would aid in their independence in performing activities of daily living. In 17% of studies, participants believed that exercise would increase their self-confidence. Fortunately, in 78% of studies, participants believed exercise would improve their health and mental well-being. Participants' demonstrated apathy for exercise in 40% of studies—either believing they would fail to achieve results or acknowledging the benefits but reporting laziness or low motivation. In 24% of studies, participants believed exercise was unnecessary for older adults and may even be harmful [6].

Future Directions

From the above study's illuminating review of elderly individuals' perspectives, a number of potential barriers are identified. These include perceptions that exercise does not improve strength, balance, and flexibility, apathy toward exercise, access difficulties such as poor transportation, and lack of adequate exercise programs and equipment. Future efforts should focus on combating these specific barriers, with the population as a whole in mind. For example, community-based educational programs can enhance understanding of the role exercise and "active aging" can have on overall health in reducing morbidity from pre-existing health conditions as well as improving overall functional status. Additionally, outreach programs to develop small class-based exercise programs can appeal to the aging population, establish positive camaraderie, and enhance attendance in ongoing exercise programs.

Future research should focus on better understanding of the health outcomes from strength and balance training as well, which are not as well-studied as aerobic activities, but may offer their own benefit profile. Community programs should look to institute both home-based and center-based efforts to appeal to a wide range of participants.

Taken together, the expected large increase in the elderly population and current barriers to adequate exercise participation in this group outline the need for a coordinated approach to promote healthy lifestyles through regular exercise. The benefits of exercise are vast, and the reward to our aging generation is immeasurable. The first prescription written for the aging athlete should be a prescription for exercise.

References

1. Lee I-M, Shiroma EJ, Lobelo F, Puska P, Blair SN, Katzmarzyk PT, et al. Effect of physical inactivity on major non-communicable diseases worldwide: an analysis of burden of disease and life expectancy. Lancet. 2012;380:219–29.
2. World Health Organization Active Ageing: a policy framework [Internet]. Aging Male. 2002. 1–37. Available from: http://www.informaworld.com/openurl?genre=article&doi=10.1080/71 3604647&magic=crossref%7C%7CD404A21C5BB053405B1A640AFFD44AE3.
3. United Nations, Department of Economic and Social Affairs PD. United Nations Economic and Social Affairs: World Population Ageing [Internet]. 2013 [cited 2017 Jan 1]. p. 114. Available from: http://www.un.org/en/development/desa/population/publications/pdf/ageing/WorldPopulationAgeing2013.pdf.
4. Bauman A, Merom D, Bull FC, Buchner DM, Fiatarone Singh MA. Updating the evidence for physical activity: summative reviews of the epidemiological evidence, prevalence, and interventions to promote "active aging". Gerontologist. 2016;56:S268–80.
5. Bouaziz W, Vogel T, Schmitt E, Kaltenbach G, Geny B, Lang PO. Health benefits of aerobic training programs in adults aged 70 and over: a systematic review. Arch Gerontol Geriatr [Internet]. 2017;69:110–27. https://doi.org/10.1016/j.archger.2016.10.012.
6. Franco MR, Tong A, Howard K, Sherrington C, Ferreira PH, Pinto RZ, et al. Older people's perspectives on participation in physical activity: a systematic review and thematic synthesis of qualitative literature. Br J Sports Med [Internet]. 2015;49:1268–76. Available from: http://bjsm.bmj.com/lookup/doi/10.1136/bjsports-2014-094015.
7. Paterson DH, Warburton DER. Physical activity and functional limitations in older adults: a systematic review related to Canada's physical activity guidelines. Int J Behav Nutr Phys Act. 2010;7:38.
8. National Council on Aging Falls Prevention Facts [Internet]. 2017. Available from: https://www.ncoa.org/news/resources-for-reporters/get-the-facts/falls-prevention-facts/.
9. Gillespie LD, Robertson MC, Gillespie WJ, Sherrington C, Gates S, Clemson LM, et al. Interventions for preventing falls in older people living in the community. Cochrane Database Syst Rev. 2012;9:CD007146.
10. McClure RJ, Turner C, Peel N, Spinks A, Eakin E, Hughes K. Population-based interventions for the prevention of fall-related injuries in older people. Cochrane Database Syst Rev. 2005;(1):CD004441.
11. Höfer S, Lim L, Guyatt G, Oldridge N. The MacNew heart disease health-related quality of life instrument: a summary. Health Qual Life Outcomes. 2004;2:3.
12. U.S. Department of Health and Human Services. 2008 Physical Activity Guidelines for Americans [Internet]. Pres. Counc. Phys. Fit. Sport. Res. Dig. 2008 [cited 2017 Jan 1]. p. 1–8. Available from: https://health.gov/paguidelines/pdf/paguide.pdf.
13. Centers for Disease Control and Prevention Stroke Facts [Internet]. 2015. Available from: https://www.cdc.gov/stroke/facts.htm.
14. Goldstein LB, Adams R, Alberts MJ, Appel LJ, Brass LM, Bushnell CD, et al. Primary prevention of ischemic stroke: a guideline from the American Heart Association/American Stroke Association stroke council: cosponsored by the atherosclerotic peripheral vascular disease interdisciplinary working group; cardiovascular nursing council. Stroke. 2006;37:1583–633.
15. Wannamethee SG, Shaper AG. Physical activity and the prevention of stroke. J Cardiovasc Risk [Internet]. 1999;6:213–6. Available from: http://journals.sagepub.com/doi/abs/10.1177/204748739900600404.
16. Angevaren M, Aufdemkampe G, Verhaar HJ, Aleman A, Vanhees L. Physical activity and enhanced fitness to improve cognitive function in older people without known cognitive impairment. Cochrane Database Syst Rev. 2008;3.
17. Blondell SJ, Hammersley-Mather R, Veerman JL. Does physical activity prevent cognitive decline and dementia?: a systematic review and meta-analysis of longitudinal studies. BMC Public Health. 2014;14:510.

18. Sofi F, Valecchi D, Bacci D, Abbate R, Gensini GF, Casini A, et al. Physical activity and risk of cognitive decline: a meta-analysis of prospective studies. J Intern Med. 2011;269:107–17.
19. Ahlskog JE, Geda YE, Graff-Radford NR, Petersen RC. Physical exercise as a preventive or disease-modifying treatment of dementia and brain aging. Mayo Clin Proc. 2011;86(9):876–84.
20. Bridle C, Spanjers K, Patel S, Atherton NM, Lamb SE. Effect of exercise on depression severity in older people: systematic review and meta-analysis of randomised controlled trials. Br J Psychiatry. 2012;201:180–5.
21. Netz Y, Wu M-J, Becker BJ, Tenenbaum G. Physical activity and psychological Well-being in advanced age: a meta-analysis of intervention studies. Psychol Aging. 2005;20(2):272–84.
22. Windle G. Exercise, physical activity and mental Well-being in later life. Rev Clin Psychol. 2014;24:319–25.
23. Windle G, Hughes D, Linck P, Russell I, Woods B. Is exercise effective in promoting mental Well-being in older age? A systematic review. Aging Ment Health. 2010;14:652–69.
24. Chodzko-Zajko WJ, Proctor DN, Singh MAF, Minson CT, Nigg CR, Salem GJ, et al. Exercise and physical activity for older adults. Med Sci Sports Exerc. 2009;41:1510–30.
25. Nelson ME, Rejeski WJ, Blair SN, Duncan PW, Judge JO, King AC, et al. Physical activity and public health in older adults. Recommendation from the American College of Sports Medicine and the American Heart Association. Circulation. 2007;116(9):1094–105.
26. Vogel T, Brechat P, Leprêtre P, Kaltenbach G, Berthel M, Lonsdorfer J. Health benefits of physical activity in older patients: a review. Int J Clin Pract. 2009;63:303–20.
27. Bouaziz W, Lang PO, Schmitt E, Kaltenbach G, Geny B, Vogel T. Health benefits of multicomponent training programmes in seniors: a systematic review. Int J Clin Pract. 2016;70:520–36.
28. Vogel T, Leprêtre P-M, Brechat P-H, Lonsdorfer E, Benetos A, Kaltenbach G, et al. Effects of a short-term personalized intermittent work exercise program (IWEP) on maximal cardio-respiratory function and endurance parameters among healthy young and older seniors. J Nutr Health Aging. 2011;15:905–11.
29. Lang PO, Bréchat PH, Vogel T, Lebreton C, Bellanger M, Rivière D, et al. Determinants of the benefits of a short-term personalized intermittent work exercise program (IWEP) among seniors: results from the CAPS program. Eur Geriatr Med. 2016;7:333–9.
30. Myers J, Prakash M, Froelicher V, Do D, Partington S, Atwood JE. Exercise capacity and mortality among men referred for exercise testing. N Engl J Med. 2002;346:793–801.
31. Cononie CC, Graves JE, Pollock ML, Ian Phillips M, Sumners C, Hagberg JM. Effect of exercise training on blood pressure in 70- to 79-yr-old men and women. Med Sci Sports Exerc [Internet]. 1991;23:505–11. Available from: https://www.scopus.com/inward/record.uri?eid=2-s2.0-0025915886&partnerID=40&md5=f47f824fdb4db4c50b27f657cc1283a2.
32. Huang G, Thompson CJ, Osness WH. Influence of a 10-week controlled exercise program on resting blood pressure in sedentary older adults. J Appl Res [Internet]. 2006;6:188–95. Available from: https://www.scopus.com/inward/record.uri?eid=2-s2.0-33751036967&partnerID=40&md5=a6fe6029e0565b83518b4ae67945f594.
33. Lee L-L, Arthur A, Avis M. Evaluating a community-based walking intervention for hypertensive older people in Taiwan: a randomized controlled trial. Prev Med (Baltimore) [Internet]. 2007;44:160–6. Available from: file://www.sciencedirect.com/science/article/pii/S0091743506003707.
34. Perini R, Fisher N, Veicsteinas A, Pendergast DR. Aerobic training and cardiovascular responses at rest and during exercise in older men and women. Med Sci Sports Exerc. 2002;34:700–8.
35. Motoyama M, Sunami Y, Kinoshita F, Kiyonaga A, Tanaka H, Shindo M, et al. Blood pressure lowering effect of low intensity aerobic training in elderly hypertensive patients. Med Sci Sports Exerc. 1998;30:818–23.
36. Vaitkevicius PV, Ebersold C, Shah MS, Gill NS, Katz RL, Narrett MJ, et al. Effects of aerobic exercise training in community-based subjects aged 80 and older: a pilot study. J Am Geriatr Soc [Internet]. 2002;50:2009–13. https://doi.org/10.1046/j.1532-5415.2002.50613.x.

37. Wanderley FAC, Oliveira J, Mota J, Carvalho J. Effects of a moderate-intensity walking program on blood pressure, body composition and functional fitness in older women: results of a pilot study. Arch Exerc Health Dis. 2010;1:50–7.
38. Kitzman DW, Brubaker PH, Herrington DM, Morgan TM, Stewart KP, Hundley WG, et al. Effect of endurance exercise training on endothelial function and arterial stiffness in older patients with heart failure and preserved ejection fraction: a randomized, controlled, single-blind trial. J Am Coll Cardiol [Internet]. 2013;62:584–92. Available from: file://www.science-direct.com/science/article/pii/S0735109713017956.
39. Sung K, Bae S. Effects of a regular walking exercise program on behavioral and biochemical aspects in elderly people with type II diabetes. Nurs Health Sci. 2012;14:438–45. https://doi.org/10.1111/j.1442-2018.2012.00690.x.
40. Coker RH, Hays NP, Williams RH, Brown AD, Freeling SA, Kortebein PM, et al. Exercise-induced changes in insulin action and glycogen metabolism in elderly adults. Med Sci Sports Exerc. 2006;38:433.
41. DiPietro L, Seeman TE, Stachenfeld NS, Katz LD, Nadel ER. Moderate-intensity aerobic training improves glucose tolerance in aging independent of abdominal adiposity. J Am Geriatr Soc [Internet]. 1998;46:875–9. https://doi.org/10.1111/j.1532-5415.1998.tb02722.x.
42. DiPietro L, Dziura J, Yeckel CW, Neufer PD. Exercise and improved insulin sensitivity in older women: evidence of the enduring benefits of higher intensity training. J Appl Physiol [Internet]. 2005;100:142 LP–149. Available from: http://jap.physiology.org/content/100/1/142.abstract.
43. Finucane FM, Sharp SJ, Purslow LR, Horton K, Horton J, Savage DB, et al. The effects of aerobic exercise on metabolic risk, insulin sensitivity and intrahepatic lipid in healthy older people from the Hertfordshire cohort study: a randomised controlled trial. Diabetologia [Internet]. 2010;53:624–31. https://doi.org/10.1007/s00125-009-1641-z.
44. Evans EM, Racette SB, Peterson LE, Villareal DT, Greiwe JS, Holloszy JO. Aerobic power and insulin action improve in response to endurance exercise training in healthy 77-87 yr olds. J Appl Physiol [Internet]. 2005;98:40–5. Available from: https://www.scopus.com/inward/record.uri?eid=2-s2.0-11144288788&doi=10.1152%2Fjapplphysiol.00928.2004&partnerID=40&md5=8809c53693ac4ba81438b3da1ea01b1b
45. World Health Organization physical activity and older adults. Glob. Strateg. Diet, Phys. Act. Heal. 2017;1.
46. Fried LP, Tangen CM, Walston J, Newman AB, Hirsch C, Gottdiener J, et al. Frailty in older adults evidence for a phenotype. J Gerontol A Biol SciMed Sci. 2001;56:M146–57.
47. Liu C-J, Latham N. Can progressive resistance strength training reduce physical disability in older adults? A meta-analysis study. Disabil Rehabil. 2011;33:87–97. http://www.who.int/dietphysicalactivity/factsheet_olderadults/en/
48. Lim SS, Vos T, Flaxman AD, Danaei G, Shibuya K, Adair-Rohani H, et al. A comparative risk assessment of burden of disease and injury attributable to 67 risk factors and risk factor clusters in 21 regions, 1990–2010: a systematic analysis for the global burden of disease study 2010. Lancet. 2013;380:2224–60.
49. Hallal PC, Andersen LB, Bull FC, Guthold R, Haskell W, Ekelund U, et al. Global physical activity levels: surveillance progress, pitfalls, and prospects. Lancet. 2012;380:247–57.

Chapter 17
Importance of Core and Gluteus Strengthening

Philip Zakko and Ron DeAngelo

Abbreviations

3DMAPS	3D Movement Analysis & Performance Systems
ITBS	Iliotibial band syndrome
PFP	Patellofemoral pain
ROM	Range of motion

Introduction

As the age of our population increases, so too does the age of our athletes. The goals of an aging athlete differ greatly from those of a young athlete. The aging athlete is not particularly concerned about performing at a professional level but is instead focused on playing their sport at the highest level their body will allow without experiencing pain or excessive labor through the activity. As such, the concept of "efficiency of movement" is very relevant to the aging athlete because it allows for full range of motion (ROM) and stability and for achieving maximum output for a given physical input.

The human body was made to move! In early civilization humans were hunters and gatherers and always on the move for 8–12 h a day. Now, society is in an age where we hunt and gather for information on a computer or television screen. At the age of five, we are told to sit down in our seats in kindergarten for half a day. Then we progress to sitting for 6–8 h right through college. A good portion of these years is also spent sitting in front of a screen watching our favorite shows and playing video games. Finally, a majority of our employment years are spent sitting for

P. Zakko
University of Pittsburgh Medical Center, Farmington, CT, USA

R. DeAngelo, MEd, CSCS, LAT, ATC, FAFS (✉)
UPMC Sports Medicine, Pittsburgh, PA, USA
e-mail: deangelors@upmc.edu

© Springer International Publishing AG, part of Springer Nature 2018
V. J. Wright, K. K. Middleton (eds.), *Masterful Care of the Aging Athlete*,
https://doi.org/10.1007/978-3-319-16223-2_17

8–12 h a day. During these times, we begin to feel cemented into postures that create "dormant butt syndrome," urinary incontinence, low back pain, and a weak core. We begin to lose ROM in our hips and our thoracic spine and can no longer move freely and efficiently.

As a result of our hectic schedules, we have a very small window to exercise. At the same time, we still like to think we are young and can just walk out the door and do our activity without properly preparing the body. After sitting or sleeping for 8 h, there is no way the body can readily be expected to perform at a high competitive level. As a consequence of dormancy, the body grows comfortable in a state that will eventually break down.

Efficiency of Movement

Efficiency of movement is achieved when the body's muscles fire efficiently to their maximum capacity. However, this is difficult to achieve because it requires necessary training of many muscle groups, which are utilized but not often realized by an athlete during activity. This is often seen in the case of an aging runner who is training for his region's marathon. His training likely focuses on running a certain distance each day and gradually increasing that distance until he reaches the marathon length. In following this routine, the aging athlete avoids targeting the most important muscle groups for efficient running: the core and gluteal muscles. His neglect of such critical muscles will likely result in injury before the marathon even begins.

During running, the gluteal muscles provide the major shock absorption when the foot lands. When properly loaded, they provide the power to drive the system. The core is the conduit in which the transfer of power of the lower extremity flows to the upper extremity. It must be noted that the inner core musculature—the pelvic floor—supersedes importance of the traditional musculature such as the transversus abdominis and oblique and back extensors. Without a strong pelvic floor, strengthening of the gluteal and outer core muscles is impossible.

There are many subtle signs of a weak pelvic floor that go undetected. The obturator internus muscle is essential for stabilization of the inner core and for various reasons can go into spasm. [CITATIONS]. The aging athlete may experience urinary leakage, which seems miniscule, when sneezing or running. Male and female may also experience frequent urination (up to 15 times a day). Often, this condition is seen as "a normal part of the aging process"; however, it is not part of the normal aging process, and health-care providers need to screen patients to treat them accordingly.

As a result of inefficient core and gluteal strength, aging athletes often experience pain and laboring during activity, which significantly impacts optimal performance. Thus, it is necessary for clinicians and physical therapists to identify patient-specific causes for inefficient movement through evaluation and clinical examinations.

Clinical Examinations

There are many physical examination tests that clinicians use to evaluate their patients for efficiency of movement. Table exams are often first used to locate an injury and potentially find a weak link that is either causing or propagating the injury. It is important to recognize that with all activity, we have to deal with the "laws of nature": gravity, ground-reactive forces, mass, and momentum. In addition, it is important to note that we move in three planes of motion: sagittal, frontal, and transverse. While table exams often succeed in isolating a particular problem, they are often ineffective in identifying which muscles in the system are causing the problem. Thus, functional tests are highly recommended as they allow a clinician to evaluate an athlete in a closed kinetic chain.

Functional tests, which exam patients motion through all three planes, are effective in replicating the examination environment in clinic as closely as possible to the patient's sport environment. As a result, functional tests allow for a more complete evaluation of a patient and can provide the clinician with knowledge about specific muscles and muscle groups that may be impacting one's performance. Nonetheless, even functional exams do not fully replicate an athlete's movement patterns during their activity.

Therefore, one must evaluate an athlete while they are performing the specific movement pattern that is creating the pain or injury. Examination would be dependent on the patient's activity and may include a gait analysis, golf swing analysis, or serving or ground stroke analysis.

Functional Examinations

The three most important areas to consider when evaluating an athlete are the foot and ankle, hip, and thoracic spine. A couple of valuable tests to assess these areas are the multidirectional single-leg squat and the thoracic spine evaluation. Additionally, a new functional test called 3D Movement Analysis & Performance Systems (or 3DMAPS) was developed by the Gray Institute to analyze all three areas simultaneously.

Multidirectional single-leg squat test: This test is designed to evaluate a person's lower extremity eccentric strength, balance, and flexibility in three planes of motion. Common compensations seen in this test are as follows:

1. Dropping of the unsupported hip (Trendelenburg's sign) indicative of a weak gluteus medius on the stabilizing leg.
2. Excessive valgus of the supporting knee, also indicative of a weak gluteus medius with possible excessive tightness in adductors or limited dorsiflexion.
3. Wobbling with lack of control of the knee on descent. This can be caused by the above issues with the addition of quadriceps and hamstring weakness.
4. Knee shaking on descent is indicative of extreme eccentric weakness in the quadriceps.

5. Consider the subtalar joint for limited range of motion and control.

The multidirectional single-leg squat test is performed on a 4–6 in. step. Patients begin by balancing on one leg. They are then instructed to reach out and down as far as possible in the sagittal plane. While maintaining control with the opposite leg, leading with the toe, patients lightly touch the floor. This is then repeated with the opposite leg which allows the clinician to assess and compare, looking for the abovementioned compensations.

Patients repeat the same movements in the frontal plane, reaching out to the side as far as possible and lightly touching the toe to the ground, and the transverse plane, reaching in a posterior lateral direction on the 5 and 7 o'clock vector with the right and left leg, respectively. In the transverse plane, it is important that the patient externally rotates at the hip of the balance leg while reaching and touching the toe to the ground lightly with the opposite foot. Repeat the exam with the opposite leg, and assess and compare, looking for compensation mechanisms.

Further testing can be performed by asking the patient to reach straight back posteriorly toward the 6 o'clock position. The patient then crosses the leg in front of or behind the balance leg at 3 or 9 o'clock, left and right leg, respectively, and finally rotating in front of the body evaluating internal rotation via the patient reaching to an 11 or 1 o'clock direction with the right or left leg, respectively.

Thoracic spine: When evaluating the thoracic spine, it is helpful to consider what osteopathic medicine describes as Type I and Type II movements that occur in this region. Simply put, Type I motion describes the thoracic spine rotating in one direction and side bending in the *opposite* direction. This test should be done standing with the hips in sync and out of sync with the torso. Golf is an example of a sport that uses Type I motion. Type II motion involves thoracic spine rotating and side bending in the *same* direction. This should also be evaluated standing with the hips in sync and out of sync with the torso. Tennis is an example of a sport that uses Type II motion.

Both motions evaluate movement in the transverse and frontal planes. It is important to note that by positioning a person in each movement pattern, you can drive them into the sagittal plane. This will allow for a 3D approach and can reveal many compensation mechanisms, which can lead to low back pain and cervical spine issues.

3D Movement Analysis & Performance System (3DMAPS): This is a newly developed movement analysis system that evaluates functional movement screen developed by the Gray Institute. It evaluates the body in its six global movement patterns, which can help provide "comprehensive, complete three dimensional assessment strategies to identify dysfunction, assess client capabilities and progress client function" [1].

When athletes—especially aging athletes—begin to experience difficulty, pain, and/or excessive labor from performing their activity, it is important to consider the strength of the core and gluteal muscles as they allow for full body stability and full ROM. Functional clinical exams are helpful in evaluating a patient's weaknesses in core and gluteal strength and can provide essential information regarding the existence of the underlying injury. 3DMAPS provides a complete evaluation of the patient by monitoring them in six global movement patterns. Next, we will examine the common injuries aging athletes experience as a result of weak core and gluteal strength.

Common Overuse Injuries Resulting from Weak Core and Gluteal Strength

Regardless of the sport, weak core and gluteal strength can lead to common injuries in the aging athlete. During certain physical activities, a deficiency in one muscle will force the body to recruit another muscle. Recruited muscles and muscle groups are typically not equipped to sustain the load and strain intended for the primary muscle group. Hence, recruited muscles are more prone to injury. A study conducted by Dehaven and Littner found that, by the seventh decade of life, the five most common athletic injuries are related to degeneration and repetitive injury [2]. In addition, a 3-year prospective evaluation of injury patterns found that overuse injuries accounted for 70% of injuries in veteran athletes (aged >60 years) but for only 41% of injuries of young athletes (aged 21–25 years) [3]. Common overuse injuries include adhesive capsulitis of the hip, low back pain, greater trochanteric bursitis, iliotibial band syndrome, piriformis syndrome, plantar fasciitis, Achilles tendonitis, and various others. One of the major causes of overuse injuries is linked to a common theme: the increasingly sedentary lifestyle of the aging population.

According to the American Heart Association, sedentary jobs have increased by 83% since 1950 with physically active jobs making up less than 20% of our workforce. This is a drastic change from 1960, where about half of the US workforce was physically active [4]. This has a profound effect on our population. It has been shown that muscle strength in sedentary individuals declines by approximately 15% per decade between the ages of 50 and 70 years and by 30% per decade after age 70. Fortunately, research shows that regular, intensive muscle exercise can minimize and/or reverse age-related declines in muscle mass [5].

Spending the majority of the day in a sedentary position results in a less mobile population due to stiffened hips and weaker muscles, especially the core and gluteal muscles. As such, when inactive individuals finally decide to begin an active lifestyle, they are at a predisposed disadvantage. They begin activity without appreciating their deficiencies in core and gluteal strength. Over time, these individuals begin to experience the common aforementioned overuse injuries. These injuries can be prevented in healthy older adults through gradual moderate- to high-intensity resistance training as seen in a study where with exercise, muscle strength increased on average from 30% (hip extensors) to 97% (hip flexors) [6].

Evidence Suggesting Core and Hip Strength Relate to Injury

To our knowledge, there are no known studies in aging athlete populations that demonstrate the relationship between hip and core strength and athletic injury. Nonetheless, there are numerous studies evaluating this relationship in younger athletes.

Souza et al. evaluated the effect of hip kinematics on patellofemoral pain (PFP) [7]. The study examined hip kinematics and activity level of hip musculature during running, a drop jump, and a step-down maneuver in 21 females with PFP and 20 pain-free controls. Averaged across all three activities, patients with PFP had increased hip internal rotation, diminished hip torque production, and significantly greater gluteus maximus recruitment [7]. It was found that increased hip internal rotation was accompanied by a decrease in hip muscle strength. Authors conclude that the increased activation of the gluteus maximus in female patients with PFP suggests that they were attempting to recruit a weakened muscle in an effort to stabilize the hip joint. PFP was also studied by Ireland et al., who found significant hip abductor and external rotator weakness in 15 female participants experiencing anterior knee pain [8]. They proposed that these weaknesses lead to uncontrolled femoral adduction and internal rotation. This, in turn, resulted in an increase in the dynamic Q angle at the knee, which is indicative of amplified stress on the patellofemoral joint.

Lee and Powers conducted a study in which they evaluated hip muscle strength with ankle biomechanics and neuromuscular activation during unipedal balance tasks [9]. The study found that females with diminished hip abductor strength exhibit increased activation of the lower leg muscles to maintain unipedal balance. This mechanism appears to be a compensatory neuromuscular response to provide ankle stability in the presence of proximal instability [10]. As an association between hip muscle strength and ankle injury has been found in a number of clinical studies, it has been suggested that such compensation places greater mechanical strain on recruited muscles resulting in overuse musculotendinous injuries [11–13].

Hip abductor weakness was also identified in 24 runners with iliotibial band syndrome (ITBS) by Fredericson et al. [14]. The authors of this study implemented a 6-week physical therapy program that emphasized hip abductor strengthening. After completing the therapy program, 22 of the 24 runners were able to return to pain-free running. From this clinical finding, the authors concluded that early recognition of deficient hip musculature strength allows for early implementation of prophylactic physical therapy and sport-specific strength training.

Leetun et al. prospectively examined differences in core stability strength measures between male and female athletes to further delineate the association between these measures and the occurrence of lower extremity injury [15]. Authors measured athlete core stability and hip strength during the preseason and tracked athletes' injury statuses through one competitive season. Lower hip strength test scores were associated with incidence of injury, with hip external rotation strength as the strongest predictor of injury [15]. Additionally, authors noted a trend that athletes who sustained an injury were found to have lower values for hip and core strength. Only hip strength tests were significantly different with hip external rotation strength as the strongest predictor of injury.

Conclusion

As a result of society's increasingly sedentary lifestyle, the number of injuries due to muscle imbalance and strength deficits is increasing. This chapter examined the importance of gluteal and core strength in order for athletes, especially the aging athlete, to perform at their optimal level and to prevent injury. Table and functional examinations were discussed with a focus on the multidirectional single-leg squat and the thoracic spine tests. It was noted that while these tests are good for effective, they are limited by not examining patients during their actual activity. The common injuries associated with a weak core and gluteal muscles are supported by an abundance of literature.

It is also important to note that the gluteal muscles are considered part of your core. In addition, the inner core, in particular the obturator internus, is a big player and often overlooked. This chapter has placed a lot of emphasis on strength, but equally as important is flexibility or normal ROM for specific joints. We should note that excessive ROM or hypermobility can be as much of a problem as hypomobility.

References

1. 3D Movement Analysis & Performance System. Functional Assessment & 3DMAPS Program. Gray Institute. Web. 20 July 2015.
2. Dehaven KE, Littner DM. Athletic injuries: comparison by age, sport, and gender. Am J Sports Med. 1986;14:218–24.
3. Kannus P, Niittymaki S, Jarvinen M, Lehto M. Sports injuries in elderly athletes: a three-year prospective, controlled study. Age Ageing. 1989;18:263–70.
4. The Price of Inactivity. The Price of Inactivity. Web. 20 July 2015. http://www.heart.org/HEARTORG/GettingHealthy/PhysicalActivity/FitnessBasics/The-Price-of-Inactivity_UCM_307974_Article.jsp
5. American College of Sports Medicine position stand: exercise and physical activity for older adults. Med Sci Sports Exerc. 1998;30:992–1008.
6. Pyka G, Lindenberger E, Charette S, Marcus R. Muscle strength and fiber adaptations to a year-long resistance training program in elderly men and women. J Gerontol. 1994;49:M22–7.
7. Souza RB, Powers CM. Differences in hip kinematics, muscle strength, and muscle activation between subjects with and without patellofemoral pain. J Orthop Sports Phys Ther. 2009;39:12–9. https://doi.org/10.2519/jospt.2009.2885.
8. Ireland ML, Wilson JD, Ballantyne BT, et al. Hip strength in females with and without patellofemoral pain. J Orthop Sports Phys Ther. 2003;33:671–6.
9. Lee S, Powers CM. Individuals with diminished hip abductor muscle strength exhibit altered ankle biomechanics and neuromuscular activation during unipedal balance tasks. Gait Posture. 2014;39(3):933–8.
10. Wubbenhorst K, Zschorlich V. Effects of muscular activation patterns on the ankle joint stabilization: an investigation under different degrees of freedom. J Electromyogr Kinesiol. 2011;21(2):340–7.
11. Kulig K, Popovich JM, Noceti-Dewit LM, Reischl SF, Kim D. Women with posterior tibial tendon dysfunction have diminished ankle and hip muscle performance. J Orthop Sports Phys Ther. 2011;41(9):687–94.
12. Friel K, McLean N, Myers C, Caceres M. Ipsilateral hip abductor weakness after inversion ankle sprain. J Athl Train. 2006;41(1):74–8.
13. Nicholas JA, Strizak AM, Veras G. A study of thigh muscle weakness in different pathological states of the lower extremity. Am J Sports Med. 1976;4(6):241–8.
14. Fredericson M, Cookingham CL, Chauhhari AM, et al. Hip abductor weakness in distance runners with iliotibial band syndrome. Clin J Sport Med. 2000;10:169–75.
15. Leetun DT, Ireland ML, Willson JD, Ballantyne BT, Davis IM. Core stability measures as risk factors for lower extremity injury in athletes. Med Sci Sports Exerc. 2004;36:926–34.

Chapter 18
Longevity and Epigenetics

James Irvine

Human Genome Project

In 2003, one of the most historic projects in modern medicine was completed, which laid out our genetic blueprint. The Human Genome Project resulted from the culmination of decades of work which includes the discovery of the double helix of deoxyribonucleic acid (DNA) and creation of laboratory tools for DNA mapping and sequencing. The human genome is made up of roughly 20,500 genes—far fewer than the initial estimates of 100,000 or more. These genes are comprised from nearly three billion A-T and G-C base pairs.

The Human Genome Project was also vital in allowing us to sequence several other genomes such as the fruit fly, mice, rats, and many others that are used to experiment and learn more about the human genome. Comparative genome analysis, revealed that 85% of the protein-coding regions are similar between mice and humans, and some genes maintain 99% of the same genetic code [2, 3]. This is important for several reasons, one being our ability to study human diseases through animal models. We have the tools available to create knockout mice which are essentially bred via genetic engineering to mimic diseases such as

J. Irvine, MD
Department of Orthopaedic Surgery, University of Pittsburgh,
Pittsburgh, PA, USA
e-mail: irvinejn@upmc.edu

© Springer International Publishing AG, part of Springer Nature 2018   213
V. J. Wright, K. K. Middleton (eds.), *Masterful Care of the Aging Athlete*,
https://doi.org/10.1007/978-3-319-16223-2_18

cystic fibrosis, DMD, and nearly any other disease which arises from an anomaly in our DNA. In addition to studying disease, it only makes sense to investigate specimens which seem to function at the highest and most optimal levels. This natural curiosity has opened up fields of research into high-level athletes, such as the "masters athlete," which is the focus of this book.

Epigenetics

Before diving into the genetic codes and protein makeup that are unique to the masters athlete, we have to take a step back and first discuss the concept of epigenetics. Epigenetics are changes that occur to our DNA or chromatin (DNA, RNA, histones, and other proteins) structure that can ultimately effect whether or not a gene can be transcribed into mRNA or not. More easily put, epigenetic changes can turn a gene "on" or "off." These modifications can include DNA methylation, histone modifications such as acetylation or methylation, and microRNA (miRNA) which are all posttranslational changes [4].

DNA methylation is a reversible process in which an enzyme known as a DNA methyltransferase (DNMT) adds a methyl group near DNA regions rich in CpG dinucleotides and is referred to as CpG islands. They normally methylate just upstream of the CpG island, which normally silences the gene [5]. This can happen in one of two ways: (1) it can have a direct effect on transcription factors or (2) recruitment of methyl-CpG-binding domain (MBD) proteins, which activate histone deacetylases (HDAC) and convert the chromatin to a repressive state [6, 7].

The other posttranslational modification targets the histones of chromatin, which are the core proteins that DNA wraps around to make up a nucleosome. Histones have a lysine-rich tail region that serves as the interactive site with histone acyltransferases (HATs) and histone deacetylases (HDACs). The function of HATs is the addition of acetyl groups which leads to activation of transcription and therefore an increase in gene expression, while HDACs remove them from DNA and effectively turn the gene off [8, 9]. Again, all of these processes are reversible mechanisms that aid in the up- and downregulation of gene expression.

MiRNAs are short sequences of noncoding RNA molecules which can silence protein translation and aid in DNA methylation and chromatin remodeling as another mechanism of epigenetic modifications of the genome [10, 11]. MiRNAs have an incredible range of function, as a single miRNA has the capability to target and regulate hundreds to even thousands of genes.

Association Between Epigenetics, Metabolic Activity, and Longevity

We will now turn our attention to the epigenetic alterations that take place in response to physical stress induced by exercise and its positive effects on metabolic states and longevity in the masters athlete. The general response to exercise is hypomethylation of several promoter regions of genes associated with metabolic activity such as peroxisome proliferator-activated receptor gamma (PPAR-γ) immediately after exercise, while others (i.e., PPAR-δ) experience a rise in expression a few hours after activity. In type 2 diabetes, PPAR-γ usually resides in a hypermethylated state, and so the exercise-induced hypomethylated form seems to provide a protective effect against type 2 diabetes [12].

Another key epigenetic mechanism that has been thoroughly investigated is the downregulation of HDAC5, one specific type of HDAC, following exercise. This is an important phenomena because HDAC5 interacts with myocyte-specific enhancer factor-2 (MEF2), which results in deacetylation of glucose transporter type 4 (GLUT4) and reduces its expression. Thus, the response to increased activity is a downregulation of HDAC5 allowing for increased levels of unbound MEF2 which can increase expression of GLUT4 in skeletal muscle and therefore regulate glucose levels and have a positive effect against type 2 diabetes [13]. Increases in MEF2 as a result of the downregulation of HDAC5 have also been associated with an increase in the number of slow-twitch muscle fibers [14].

The other epigenetic modifier includes miRNAs which are tissue-specific regulators. Studies have shown that both acute high-intensity aerobic exercise and distance training have profound impact on several miRNAs with the net effect being a decrease in their expression. This has the ability to alter genes involved in the transcription machinery as well as ones directly involved in muscle metabolism resulting in an increase in expression of lipid oxidation and mitochondrial enzymes [15]. MiRNAs have been implicated in the remodeling of skeletal muscle to include regulatory mechanisms involving angiogenesis which is an important component of muscle perfusion and oxidative phosphorylation associated with aerobic exercise [16].

These epigenetic processes are present throughout life and play a direct role in the aging process to include the development of pathological diseases associated with the elderly. At the genomic level, aging is directly related to the shortening of telomeres, which are the ends of chromosomes that protect it from deterioration. Unfortunately, telomeres are shortened after each cell division, which will eventually reach cellular senescence. The telomere regions themselves are believed to be comprised of noncoding RNAs which can interact with and regulate telomere length. Research has shown that exercise upregulates telomerase activity and can provide a protective effect to the cell by maintenance of telomere length [17].

The benefits of exercise demonstrated by the masters athlete is not limited to skeletal muscle but may also preserve and help maintain other vital structures to include neural tissue. Specifically, recent research into sirtuins, a family of proteins linked to cell survival, has been implicated in the longevity of neural tissue and may protect against neurodegenerative diseases [18]. A healthy mind is an essential component of healthy aging and longevity, so it only seems natural that the biochemical alterations which result from physical activity not only build and maintain skeletal muscle tissue but also preserve brain function and possibly avoid cognitive decline.

References

1. https://www.genome.gov/10001772/all-about-the--human-genome-project-hgp/
2. https://www.genome.gov/12011238/an-overview-of-the-human-genome-project/
3. http://www.genome.gov/10001345/
4. Eccleston A, DeWitt N, Gunter C, Marte B, Nath D. Epigenetics. Nat Insight. 2007;447(7143):396–440.
5. Doi A, Park IH, Wen B, et al. Differential methylation of tissue- and cancer-specific CpG island shores distinguishes human induced pluripotent stem cells, embryonic stem cells and fibroblasts. Nat Genet. 2009;41(12):1350–3.
6. Feng J, Fouse S, Fan G. Epigenetic regulation of neural gene expression and neuronal function. Pediatr Res. 2007;61(5 Pt 2):58R–63R.
7. Phillips T. The role of methylation in gene expression. Nat Educ. 2008;1(1):116.
8. McGee SL, Hargreaves M. Histone modifications and exercise adaptations. J Appl Physiol. 2011;110(1):258–63.
9. McKinsey TA, Zhang CL, Olson EN. Control of muscle development by dueling HATs and HDACs. Curr Opin Genet Dev. 2001;11(5):497–504.
10. Baek D, Villen J, Shin C, et al. The impact of microRNAs on protein output. Nature. 2008;455(7209):64–71.
11. Baltimore D, Boldin MP, O'Connell RM, et al. MicroRNAs: new regulators of immune cell development and function. Nat Immunol. 2008;9(8):839–45.
12. Barres R, Yan J, Egan B, et al. Acute exercise remodels promoter methylation in human skeletal muscle. Cell Metab. 2012;15(3):405–11.
13. McGee SL, Hargreaves M. Exercise and skeletal muscle glucose transporter 4 expression: molecular mechanisms. Clin Exp Pharmacol Physiol. 2006;33(4):395–9.
14. Potthoff MJ, Wu H, Arnold MA, et al. Histone deacetylase degradation and MEF2 activation promote the formation of slow-twitch myofibers. J Clin Invest. 2007;117(9):2459–67.
15. Keller P, Vollaard NB, Gustafsson T, et al. A transcriptional map of the impact of endurance exercise training on skeletal muscle phenotype. J Appl Physiol. 2011;110(1):46–59.
16. Fernandes T, Magalhaes FC, Roque FR, et al. Exercise training prevents the microvascular rarefaction in hyper-tension balancing angiogenic and apoptotic factors: role of microRNAs-16, -21, and -126. Hypertension. 2012;59(2):513–20.
17. Werner C, Furster T, Widmann T, et al. Physical exercise prevents cellular senescence in circulating leukocytes and in the vessel wall. Circulation. 2009;120(24):2438–47.
18. Pallas M, Verdaguer E, Tajes M, et al. Modulation of sirtuins: new targets for antiageing. Recent Pat CNS Drug Discov. 2008;3(1):61–9.

Index

U
Ultrasound
  osteoporosis, 10
  sarcopenia, 12
Unicompartmental knee arthroplasty
       (UKA), 82
  indications, 176
  Knee Society survey, 177, 178
  medial/lateral tibiofemoral
       compartment, 176
  patellofemoral arthroplasty, 177
  survival rate, 177
US Preventive Services Task Force
       (USPSTF), 10

V
Vascular changes, 13
Vegetables, 32
Verbal learning and memory test (VLMT), 198
Veterans Affairs system, 48

Victorian Institute of Sport Assessment-
       Achilles (VISA-A) questionnaire,
       146, 147
Viscosupplementation
  composition, 65
  efficacy, 65
  hyaluronate, 65
  mechanism of action, 65
  side effects, 66
  synovial fluid, 65
Visual analog score (VAS), 146–149
Vitamin D, 40
Volar plating, 139

W
Walch classification, 120, 121
Whey protein, 41
Wisconsin card-sorting test, 198
wnt pathway, 49
World Health Organization (WHO), 10, 25